
Jeff May's Healthy Home Tips

Jeff May's

HEALTHY

HOME

TIPS

THE JOHNS HOPKINS UNIVERSITY PRESS

Baltimore

A WORKBOOK
for DETECTING,
DIAGNOSING,
& ELIMINATING

Pesky Pests,
Stinky Stenches,
Musty Mold, and Other
Aggravating Home Problems

Jeffrey C. May &
Connie L. May

Note: The authors are neither physicians nor attorneys and are not attempting to provide medical or legal advice. The services of a competent professional should be obtained whenever medical, legal, or other specific advice is needed. Neither the publisher nor the authors make any warranty, either express or implied, regarding the recommendations or practices described in this book, nor do they assume liability for any consequences arising from the use of the content of this book.

The Johns Hopkins University Press
2715 North Charles Street
Baltimore, Maryland 21218-4363
www.press.jhu.edu

Library of Congress Cataloging-in-Publication Data
May, Jeffrey C.
    Jeff May's healthy home tips : a workbook for detecting, diagnosing, and eliminating pesky pests, stinky stenches, musty mold, and other aggravating home problems / Jeffrey C. May and Connie L. May.
        p. cm.
Includes index.
ISBN-13: 978-0-8018-8845-8 (pbk. : alk. paper)
ISBN-10: 0-8018-8845-X (pbk. : alk. paper)
1. Housing and health — Popular works. I. May, Connie L. II. Title.
RA770.M39 2008
613'.5 — dc22   2007040653

A catalog record for this book is available from the British Library.

Illustrations on pages 27, 28, 29, 35, 36, 37, 68, 91, 100, 114, 134, 136, and 139 are © Tom Feiza, Mr. Fix-It, Inc., author of *How to Operate Your Home,* and are reproduced with permission.

Special discounts are available for bulk purchases of this book. For more information, please contact Special Sales at 410-516-6936 or specialsales@press.jhu.edu.

The Johns Hopkins University Press uses environmentally friendly book materials, including recycled text paper that is composed of at least 30 percent post-consumer waste, whenever possible. All of our book papers are acid-free, and our jackets and covers are printed on paper with recycled content.

Contents

Jeff May's Healthy Home Tips

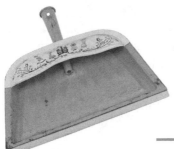

Introduction

JEFF'S OPENING GEMS

For many years people have been concerned about outdoor contaminants, like smoke billowing from power-plant chimneys, smog in city air, and chemicals discharged into our rivers or buried in the soil. But more and more people are now realizing that pollutants indoors also may be damaging to health.

When we discuss these indoor pollutants, we are talking about "indoor air quality," or IAQ. We know that outdoor air moves because we can feel wind on our skin, but air also flows within buildings, and these gentle "breezes" can carry irritants, allergens, and contaminants that either enter a building from the exterior or are generated by sources within. Just by breathing, our lungs and bodies are exposed to many of these substances. Some of the substances are gases or vapors, and others are particulates (airborne particles).

The list of invisible junk floating in the air in buildings, including our homes, is remarkably long and includes:

- Mold spores
- Bacteria
- Yeast
- Mite droppings and body parts
- Fragments of spider droppings
- Cat and dog dander
- Wool dander shed by some wool carpets
- Solvents from paints, caulks, and adhesives
- Chemicals and particles emitted by copiers and printers

- Chemicals emitted by new synthetic carpeting
- Carbon monoxide and soot from heating and cooling equipment
- Formaldehyde from furnishings and construction materials
- Carbon dioxide in our breath
- Odors from people's bodies (some emitted continuously, others intermittently!)
- Cigarette smoke
- Fragrances and solvents from cleaning compounds
- Soot and fragrances from jar candles
- Smoke from wood stoves and fireplaces

Any one of these substances can cause health symptoms. My job as an IAQ consultant is to try to find conditions indoors that may be causing or contributing to people's health problems.

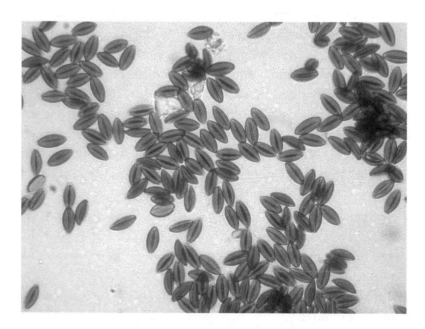

These spores came from mold growing on a wood baseboard hidden in a corner behind the edge of a carpet. Moisture fueling the mold growth came from a crack in a brick exterior wall that faced the direction of prevailing rainstorm winds. *May Indoor Air Investigations LLC*

Some of the stories I hear about spaces that make people feel sick sound like Connie's unpublished fiction, but they really happened. Here are a few examples:

- The children's bath time that nearly suffocated their mother.
- The unfinished basement that smelled like a dead fish.
- The bedroom that made a man's right lung vibrate.
- The den that gave its owner a runny nose.

Each of these situations developed for a reason.

• *The nearly lethal bath time.* The woman had two small children. Sometimes when she bathed them in the tub, her mouth and face swelled. Her windpipe also swelled, blocking her breathing. She was hospitalized several times before calling me in to see if something in her house was causing her symptoms. I found *Aspergillus* mold growing in the dust in the basement playroom carpet. When the children played on the carpet, they got *Aspergillus* spores in their hair. Then the woman was exposed to the spores when she shampooed her children's hair. She was severely allergic to this kind of mold, so her symptoms were extreme and frightening. After professional remediators removed the basement carpet and installed a vinyl floor, the woman was once again able to enjoy bath time with her children.

• *The dead fish odor.* In a basement light, a plastic surround insulated the metal bulb socket. This plastic was decomposing, resulting in a smell reminiscent of dead fish. The stinky fixture was removed and replaced with one that had a porcelain socket insulator, and the stench never returned.

• *The vibrating lung.* Wind outside caused changes in air pressure in the attic. When the attic air pressure increased, it pushed against and slightly depressed the newly laid attic floor. As the floor was deflected down, the ceiling of the bedroom below was also pushed down, resulting in an increase in the air pressure in the room. (The same amount of air took up less space.) When the attic air pressure decreased, the attic floor rose and the ceiling below rose with it. The air pressure in the bedroom then decreased. (The same amount of air took up more space.) When he was in bed, the man experienced these wind-driven air-pressure changes in his right lung as vibrations, which kept him awake much of the night. He put books on the attic floor, which reduced its movements, and he overcame his insomnia. (When this man first called me and described the feeling he had in his right lung, I wondered about his sanity, but working with him taught me to always believe the client.)

• *The runny nose.* After he retired, the owner of the house, a surgeon, was hoping to spend more time in his den, which contained a large fish tank. The man complained that his nose dripped whenever he was in the room. "If I'd had this condition when I was working," he told me, "I could never have been a surgeon."

I found dust mites crawling all over the top and underside of the tank cover. Why were they there? When the man sprinkled fish food into the water, some of the flakes stuck to the underside of the tank cover where moisture had condensed. Dust mites require moisture and love fish flakes. In fact, that's what I feed my dust mite colony.

CONNIE'S COMMENTS

He really does sometimes keep a dust mite colony. (Thankfully, they seldom survive long.) He looks at the creatures under his microscope. He also puts petri dishes under spider webs to catch the spider's droppings so he can examine them under his microscope. He's a little odd, but endearing in his own way!

When the man fed his fish, he opened and closed the tank cover, and that's when dust containing mite droppings and body parts spread into the air. Not surprisingly, he was allergic to dust mites. He had the cover of the tank and all of the dust in the den cleaned up, and his den difficulties evaporated.

As you can see, figuring out the cause of each of these problems led to a cure. You may be looking for a cure because you or someone in your family is experiencing health symptoms in a particular room and feels better when away from the space. People often ask me if conditions where they live or work may be causing them to cough, sneeze, or wheeze. I believe that the answer to this question is "yes"; otherwise, I wouldn't be writing this book.

If you are suffering health symptoms that you believe may be worse in-doors, keep a written record of your symptoms (when you experience them, where and what is going on in the space at the time) and share them with your physician or with a physician who is knowledgeable about the impact the indoor environment can have on human health. Wear a respirator or a NIOSH (National Institute of Occupational Safety and Health) N95 mask if you enter a musty-smelling or moldy area. Carry several such masks with you when you travel.

But even if you or someone in your family is not experiencing any health symptoms indoors, this book will help you maintain a "healthy home" by keeping your indoor air clean. There are steps you can take to eradicate the potential sources of indoor air quality problems (listed in the book as "Dos") and actions to avoid taking because they may cause IAQ problems (listed as "Don'ts"). Dos and Don'ts that are primarily relevant to those who are sensitized — reactive to certain substances in the environment — are placed at the end of Dilemma sections where relevant, under the heading "For People with Allergies, Asthma, or Environmental Sensitivities."

Part I deals with mold. Part II discusses other sources of IAQ problems. Throughout the book I add some of the questions people have asked me or summaries of case studies from my work. There is also space for you to record your own observations and concerns, as well as keep track of the steps you've taken. Be as detailed as you can, because your record-keeping can guide you in your efforts to improve the quality of your indoor environment. Lastly, I include relevant resources at the end of many of the sections, and there is a list of additional resources at the end of the book.

This book is not intended to offer an all-encompassing account of the causes of and possible cures for poor indoor air quality. After all, this is my fourth book on the subject, and I feel as if I still have more to say! This book is a good place to start, though, and you can refer to the other three books I've published[*] for more detailed discussions and information about indoor air quality in residential and other types of buildings, including offices and schools.

---

[*] *My House Is Killing Me! The Home Guide for Families with Allergies and Asthma; The Mold Survival Guide: For Your Home and for Your Health;* and *My Office Is Killing Me! The Sick Building Survival Guide.*

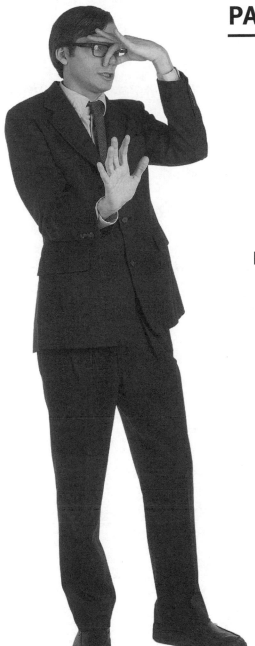

PART I

Mold, Mildew, and You

Is that black fuzzy stuff mold? If so, why it is growing there? How do I get rid of it? Will it grow back? Answer these questions and you will make major progress in your battle against mold.

JEFF'S GEMS

Mold is part of the Kingdom of Fungi. In Part I, I discuss two categories of fungi:

1. *Fleshy macrofungi, which grow fruiting bodies we call mushrooms or toadstools.*
2. *Powdery microfungi, or what laymen call mold or mildew, which produce microscopic spores all along the surface of the fungal growth.*

Macrofungi can cause structural damage to the wood in buildings if the fungal growth is extensive enough. But microfungi, with only a few exceptions, do not pose structural threats to buildings. They do, however, produce spores that can negatively affect human health. Mildew growth indoors is a potential health hazard.

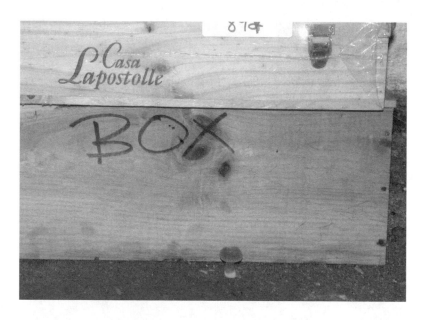

Steady water in the form of a fine mist coming from a minute pin-hole leak in a pipe sprinkled the soil for years around a box in a wine cellar. A fungus decayed soil debris and the bottom of the box and produced this little mushroom. *May Indoor Air Investigations LLC*

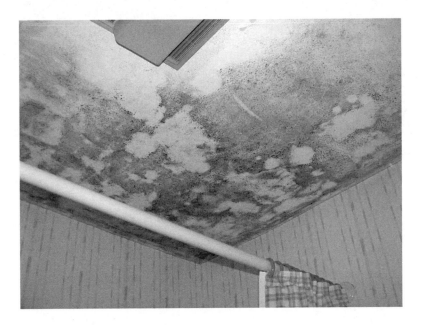

Moisture from many long, hot showers led to this nightmarish microfungal growth on a drywall bathroom ceiling. Surface dust and drywall paper served as nutrients for the mold. *May Indoor Air Investigations LLC*

CONNIE'S COMMENTS

He does tend to lecture, doesn't he? But he has some relevant information to share.

RELEVANT RESOURCES

Websites with Information about Mold

www.iaqa.org/mold＿resources＿links.htm: The Indoor Air Quality Association, Inc. (IAQA)'s "Mold Resources Links" Website.

www.cdc.gov/mold/: The Centers for Disease Control and Prevention (CDC) "Environmental Hazards and Health Effects — Mold" Website.

www.cdc/gov/health/mold.html: The CDC's "Mold" Website.

www.doh.wa.gov/ehp/ts/IAQ/got＿mold.html: The Washington State Department of Health, Division of Environmental Health, Office of Environmental Health and Safety's "Gold Mold? Frequently Asked Questions about Mold" Website.

www.epa.gov/mold/moldresources.html: The U.S. Environmental Protection Agency (EPA) "Mold Resources" Website.

www.moldtips.com: The National Association of Home Builders (NAHB) "Household Mold" Website.

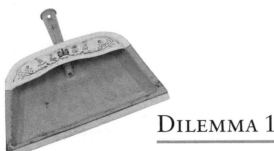

Dilemma 1

Mold, Inside and Out

One of your first jobs is to try to figure out whether there is any visible mold in your home. Musty odors can be a sign of mold growth, but such odors may also indicate a concealed infestation of shrews or mice. (See Part II, Dilemma 3E, "Pets and Pests.") Mildew (microfungal growth) is sometimes hard to see. Hold a bright flashlight almost parallel to the leg of a table or chair, or to the lower few feet of a wall in a cold closet or in a finished basement room. If you see fuzzy white, light yellow, or pale blue-green oval spots, you are probably looking at mold colonies. If you touch the spots, mold spores may become airborne. (Refer to Part I, Dilemma 2, "Confirmation and Remediation.")

Your second job is to understand the conditions conducive to mold growth so you can work to change those conditions. This section of the book will help you to identify mold growth inside, get rid of it as safely as possible, and reduce the chances that it will grow again.

Begin with the checklist on page 12.

JEFF'S GEMS

Mildew can grow within 24 to 48 hours whenever moisture (from leaks, spills, high relative humidity, or condensation), air and food sources (skin scales, wood, and starch in drywall, cardboard, and paper, among others) are present. You can't get rid of air, and biodegradable dust is everywhere. You can, however, minimize moisture, which is the key to preventing mildew growth.

CONNIE'S COMMENTS

Don't be discouraged. You really can minimize the chances of mildew growth if you follow Jeff's advice.

A. MY BASEMENT

_____ Rooms above my basement or crawl space smell musty.

_____ My basement or crawl space smells musty.

_____ I think I see mold on the basement walls.

_____ Mold grows on possessions stored in the basement. (Refer to Part I, Dilemma 2B, "Cleaning It Up Myself," and 2C, "Hiring Professionals to Remediate.")

_____ Spending time in our finished basement makes me or someone in my family feel sick.

_____ I have other concerns. _____

_____

_____

Conditions in My Basement or Crawl Space

_____ My basement and/or crawl space has a dirt floor.

_____ The ceiling in my basement and/or crawl space has exposed fiberglass insulation.

_____ I get water in my basement or crawl space.

If so, when? _____

Where? _____

_____

_____ Do you dehumidify your basement in summer?

With a portable dehumidifier that needs to be emptied? _____

With a dehumidifier placed above a sink or attached to a condensate pump that drains into a sink or to the exterior? _____

_____ My basement has been finished into rooms.

What are the rooms used for? _____

_____

_____

_____ Do you have rugs or wall-to-wall carpeting in the basement?

_____ Do you keep your finished basement warm in winter?

If so, at what temperature?

During the day _____

At night _____

When you are away from the house for several days or longer

_____

JEFF'S GEMS

As far as the flow of air is concerned, your crawl space or basement is part of your home. Surfaces in these below-grade (below ground level) spaces should be as clean as surfaces in the rest of the house, or mold spores or other allergens or irritants can move upward on airflows into the rooms above.

➤ A Crawl Space under the House

Cleanliness

Do

_____ Install lighting so you can check for

  _____ mold growth

  _____ condensation

  _____ plumbing leaks under tubs, stall showers, and sinks

  _____ fallen and shredded insulation — usually a sign of pest infestation, which can smell like mold. (See Part II, Dilemma 3E, "Pets and Pests.")

_____ Have plumbing leaks repaired.

_____ Paint the concrete floor and walls for easier cleaning; use a paint suitable for concrete.

_____ If possible, HEPA vacuum (use a vacuum cleaner with high efficiency particulate arrestance filtration) the concrete floor and walls once a year.

_____ Isolate a moldy or musty-smelling crawl space from the basement and habitable spaces above by closing windows and access openings.

CONNIE'S COMMENTS

One homeowner e-mailed us, "My crawl space stinks but I'm afraid to go down there because it's dark." This man's fear of his dark and smelly crawl space explains in part why crawl spaces can be such a problem.

_____ Have a moldy or musty-smelling crawl space professionally remediated. (See Part I, Dilemma 2C, "Hiring Professionals to Remediate.")

Dehumidification

Do

_____ Dehumidify during the warmer months.
　　_____ Seal the exterior vents of an attached, healthy (non-moldy) crawl space.
　　_____ Leave the crawl space open to the dehumidified basement.
　　_____ If there is no basement, dehumidify the crawl space itself. (See "Dehumidification," in the "Unfinished Basement" section that follows.)

JEFF'S GEMS

Many building codes for new construction still require that crawl spaces be open to the exterior and ventilated. I don't agree. In most climates, ventilating a crawl space to the exterior can introduce humid air into the space and fuel mold growth within. Some building codes are changing, however, and now allow unventilated crawl spaces in new construction. See www.crawlspaces .org.

_____ Keep the relative humidity (RH) at no more than 50%.

_____ Monitor the RH with a hygrometer, available online and in many building supply and hardware stores.

CONNIE'S COMMENTS

Let's slow down a little here, Jeff, and explain what the term "relative humidity" means. It's time for a brief lecture.

JEFF'S GEMS

Relative humidity (RH) is a measure of how much water vapor air at a given temperature is holding, versus how much water vapor that air at the same temperature can hold. If air is at 60% relative humidity, it has 40% more capacity to hold water vapor until it reaches the saturation point (100% RH), when moisture begins to condense on cooler surfaces. Cooler air has a reduced capacity to hold water vapor. If we take that air with 60% RH and cool it, the RH will rise even though we are not introducing more water vapor into the air.

Air does not always have the same temperature throughout an indoor space. Air next to cool basement walls or near the slab (the concrete foundation floor) is usually cooler than air at eye level in the middle of the basement. This cooler air has a higher relative humidity. As the RH rises above 75%, some molds can grow on surface dust as well as on dust captured in carpeting and fiberglass insulation.

A Dirt Floor

Do

_____ If there is sufficient clearance, cover a dirt floor with crushed stone, a vapor barrier (a water-impermeable plastic), and concrete.

_____ If there is insufficient clearance for crushed stone, a vapor barrier, and concrete, consider installing Neutocrete (an insulating concrete material that can be pumped into spaces with low clearance) over the dirt (www.neutocrete.com).

_____ If neither concrete nor Neutocrete is an option, keep the soil free of biodegradable materials such as cardboard and wood, and cover the soil completely with a heavy vapor barrier, such as plastic laminated to mesh, fastened securely to the foundation walls.

    _____ When access to plumbing, electrical, or mechanical equipment is necessary, create treated-wood "walkways" on top of an exposed vapor barrier to prevent foot traffic from damaging the plastic.

_____ Whenever potentially moldy soil is disturbed, the work should be done under containment, and the person doing the work should have respiratory protection (should at least wear a two-strap mask with a National Institute of Occupational Safety and Health — NIOSH — rating of N95).

JEFF'S GEMS

To set up containment, the work space should be isolated from the rest of the house. Doors and other openings leading from the basement or crawl space to the house should be closed and covered with plastic. A fan should be used on an exhaust setting to blow air out of the basement or crawl space. This reduces the work space's air pressure (creating "negative pressure"), so air flows through gaps and cracks into the basement or crawl space from the habitable spaces above, rather than vice versa.

CONNIE'S COMMENTS

Choose your contractor carefully. One client asked her contractor if he "had negative pressure while working." The contractor thought the client was re-

ferring to his boss and replied "yes," but he never used the exhaust fans he should have used. Needless to say, the house was full of contaminated dust after the work was done.

Don't

_____ Have a dirt floor in a crawl space.

Insulation

Do

_____ If building codes require fiberglass insulation in the ceiling, cover the insulation with a noncombustible material such as DensShield (fiberglass-backed drywall) which has been pre-painted.

_____ If allowed to do so by building codes, install at least one-inch thick, foil-laminated solid-sheet foam insulation against the foundation walls rather than fiberglass insulation in the ceiling structure.

_____ If required to do so by codes, cover the foam insulation with a noncombustible material such as painted DensShield.

_____ Leave the last inch or two at the top of the foundation wall uncovered so that you or a professional can inspect for termite activity (mud tubes going up the foundation wall).

Don't

_____ Leave fiberglass ceiling or wall insulation exposed or open to the exterior. (See Part II, Dilemma 3E, "Pets and Pests.")

Storage

Do

_____ Store personal possessions on metal or plastic shelves several inches above the concrete floor and eighteen inches away from uninsulated foundation walls.

Don't

_____ Store possessions in a crawl space with a dirt floor, even if the floor is covered with a vapor barrier.

➤ An Unfinished Basement
  (a basement with bare foundation walls and floor)

Cleanliness

Do

_____ Paint the concrete floor and walls for easier cleaning; use a paint suitable for concrete.

_____ HEPA vacuum the floor and walls, including the top of the foundation, once or twice a year to maintain cleanliness.

_____ Isolate a moldy or musty-smelling basement from habitable spaces by closing the door and access openings leading from the basement to the rooms above.

_____ Have a moldy or musty-smelling basement professionally remediated. (See Part I, Dilemma 2C, "Hiring Professionals to Remediate.")

_____ Use a rubber mat instead of a rug for comfort in the laundry area.

Don't

_____ Let leaves and debris collect under the basement stairs.

_____ Place a rug on the concrete floor.

_____ Allow workers to saw wood in the basement, especially if you have exposed fiberglass insulation in the basement ceiling. Fiberglass captures dust, including sawdust, which can then become moldy if the relative humidity is high enough — more than 75–80%.

Dehumidification

Do

_____ Dehumidify during the warmer months.

_____ Keep the relative humidity (RH) at no more than 50%.

_____ Monitor the RH with a hygrometer, available online and in many building supply and hardware stores.

_____ Buy only a dehumidifier with a filter of MERV-7 or better, to prevent dust from collecting on the cooling coil and then getting moldy. (MERV stands for "minimum efficiency reporting value.")

_____ Consider using a larger-capacity machine such as a Therma-Stor Santa Fe (www.thermastor.com), which will work efficiently in cooler basement temperatures and comes equipped with a MERV-11 filter.

_____ Drain the dehumidifier into a sink or use a condensate pump that discharges into a sink or to the exterior.

_____ Keep the dehumidifier free of dust and the cooling coil clean.

Don't

_____ Install a so-called "dehumidifier" that only exhausts basement air to the exterior.

_____ Operate a dehumidifier when doing dusty work like sawing wood unless the dehumidifier has MERV-7 or better filtration.

A Dirt Floor

Do

_____ Cover a dirt floor with crushed stone, a vapor barrier, and concrete.

_____ If you cannot install concrete now, clear the soil of biodegradable materials and cover the soil completely with a heavy vapor barrier fastened securely to the foundation walls. (See www.crawlspaces .org.)

     _____ Where access to plumbing, electrical, or mechanical equipment is necessary, create treated-wood "walkways" on top of an exposed vapor barrier to prevent foot traffic from ripping holes in the plastic.

_____ Whenever potentially moldy soil is disturbed, the work should be done under containment, and whoever is doing the work should have respiratory protection (should at least wear a two-strap mask with a NIOSH rating of N95).

Don't

_____ Have a dirt floor in an unfinished basement.

Human Activity

Don't

_____ Exercise in a musty-smelling basement.

_____ Let children play in a moldy or musty-smelling basement or on an old basement carpet.

Insulation

Do

_____ If building codes require fiberglass insulation in a basement ceiling, cover the insulation with a noncombustible material such as DensShield (fiberglass-backed drywall) which has been pre-painted.

_____ If allowed to do so by building codes, install at least one-inch thick, foil-laminated solid-sheet foam insulation against the foundation walls rather than fiberglass insulation in the ceiling structure.

    _____ If required to do so by codes, cover the foam insulation with a noncombustible material such as painted DensShield (fiberglass-backed drywall).

    _____ Leave the last inch or two at the top of the foundation uncovered so that you or a professional can inspect for termite activity (mud tubes going up the foundation wall).

Don't

_____ Leave fiberglass ceiling or wall insulation exposed. (See Part II, Dilemma 3E, "Pets and Pests.")

JEFF'S GEMS

In approximately one-third of the houses I've investigated containing exposed fiberglass insulation in an unfinished basement, the fiberglass was infested with mold. Even if the fiberglass was supposedly clean, I found mold flourishing in the captured dust. More often than not, mold-eating mites were also present, foraging on the mold. Exposed fiberglass insulation in a crawl space ventilated to the exterior and with a dirt floor is often similarly infested, because damp outdoor air flowing into the crawl space causes excess relative humidity.

And unless an unfinished crawl space or basement is being adequately *dehumidified in the warmer, more humid months, personal possessions placed directly on a cool concrete floor or in contact with the cool foundation wall can become peppered with mold growth.*

Moisture Control

Do

_____ Determine the source of the moisture condensing on surfaces. (Water can evaporate from one place and condense on a remote place where the temperature is lower.)

    _____ If there is a pipe leak, repair it.

    _____ If the relative humidity is higher than 50%, dehumidify.

    _____ Keep windows and the door or bulkhead closed to prevent the entry of moist air.

    _____ Have an inside door leading to the bulkhead to minimize the infiltration of moist air (as well as prevent pest entry; see Part II, Dilemma 3E, "Pets and Pests").

_____ Cover cold water pipes with tubular foam insulation to prevent them from "sweating" (condensation of moisture) in humid weather.

_____ Keep any sump pump low enough to prevent overflow from the sump during heavy rain, but not so low that the sump is submerged under the water table and runs almost continuously.

    _____ If flooding and power outages are common in your area, consider installing a floor water alarm and a battery-operated high-water alarm for the sump, along with a battery-operated back-up sump pump.

    _____ If you have a central alarm system, connect the floor water alarm to it.

Storage

Do

_____ Store personal possessions on metal or plastic shelves, several inches above the concrete floor and eighteen inches away from uninsulated foundation walls.

_____ Seal clothing in plastic bins to protect items from mildew. (Make sure the clothing is completely dry first.)

_____ If you must keep shelving against a foundation wall, place foil-laminated sheet foam insulation between the shelving and the foundation.

CONNIE'S COMMENTS

Rolling shelves are great for storage as long as there is a concrete floor. (No shelves on a dirt floor, please!)

Don't

_____ Store possessions in a basement with a dirt floor, even if the floor is covered with a vapor barrier.

_____ Store cardboard boxes on dirt or concrete.

_____ Keep vast collections of personal possessions in unfinished basements. (You can't clean what you can't get to.)

_____ Install wooden storage benches or a wooden workbench against an uninsulated foundation wall.

► A Finished Basement
   (a basement that contains rooms with walls and floors)

Cleanliness

Do

_____ HEPA vacuum (use a vacuum cleaner with high efficiency particulate arrestance filtration) and dust surfaces on the same schedule as you vacuum and clean the rest of your house (ideally a minimum of once a week).

_____ Keep baseboard heating convectors dust-free with an annual cleaning.

_____ Clean dirty baseboard convectors by removing the front cover and HEPA vacuuming the fins.

_____ If all the dust between the fins cannot be removed with a HEPA vacuum, use steam from a steam-vapor machine to clean the fins.

JEFF'S GEMS

Steam vapor machines are available in some building supply stores and on-line. (See www.vaporcleanproducts.com and www.allergybuyersclub.com.) This device is not what people commonly refer to as a steam cleaner, which uses liquid water for cleaning. A steam vapor machine looks like a vacuum cleaner, but the canister is filled with water and only steam comes out of the cleaning head. Be sure to follow manufacturer's directions for safe use. For fabrics, rugs, cushions, and other fleecy materials, spot check an area of the material you intend to treat with steam vapor first, to be sure the steam won't cause any damage. Metal surfaces can be safely treated with steam vapor.

_____ Have a moldy or musty-smelling crawl space professionally remediated. (See Part I, Dilemma 2, "Confirmation and Remediation.")

Dehumidification

Do

_____ Dehumidify all spaces during the warmer months.

    _____ Keep the relative humidity (RH) at no more than 50%.

    _____ Monitor the RH with a hygrometer, available online and in many building supply and hardware stores.

_____ Keep connecting doors (even to closets) open to dehumidify each space separately, or have louvered doors installed.

_____ Use a ducted dehumidifier if air in a central dehumidified space cannot flow to all areas or rooms.

_____ Since dehumidifier coils can get moldy, buy only a dehumidifier with a MERV-7 or better filter. (MERV stands for "minimum efficiency reporting value.")

_____ Consider using a larger-capacity machine such as a Therma-Stor Santa Fe (www.thermastor.com), which will work efficiently in cooler basement temperatures.

_____ Drain a dehumidifier into a sink or use a condensate pump that discharges into a sink or to the exterior.

_____ Keep a dehumidifier free of dust and the cooling coil clean.

Don't

_____ Operate a dehumidifier in the heating season.

_____ Operate a dehumidifier if there is ice on the coil. (This means that the air is too cold to dehumidify efficiently.)

_____ Operate a dehumidifier if the coil is dirty.

_____ Operate a dehumidifier when you are sawing wood, because the machine will draw in sawdust.

_____ Allow isolated spaces (rooms with closed doors, a cabinet under the basement stairs, a closet) to be without dehumidification.

_____ Install a so-called "dehumidifier" that only exhausts basement air to the exterior.

Finishing the Basement

Do

_____ Use sheet-foam insulation on the foundation behind finished walls rather than fiberglass insulation between the wall studs. (Sheet-foam insulation doesn't trap dust or water.)

_____ Leave a narrow walking space between the back of a finished wall and the foundation, so you can inspect for pests or leaks and mop up after a flood.

    _____ If you cannot afford to lose the space, use metal studs, but leave a one-inch gap between the foundation and the studs and use spray-foam insulation (such as Icynene or Corbond) between and behind the studs.

_____ Install a ceramic tile or vinyl floor.

    _____ Use area rugs if you want a softer feel underfoot.

_____ For a more even distribution of heat, choose hot-water or electric baseboard heat or electric radiant heat, rather than hot-air heat.

Don't

_____ Install wall-to-wall carpeting in a below-grade (below ground level) space.

_____ Install wood framing on concrete to create a raised floor.

JEFF'S GEMS

It's often tempting to install a raised wooden floor on joists over a concrete slab. This type of construction leaves a concealed space that is almost always inaccessible, however, and if there are moisture sources present in the space, mold growth or decay can spread unseen. Particularly if insulated with fiberglass, such spaces can become rodent hotels. (See Part II, Dilemma 3E, "Pets and Pests.") If you insist on having a raised floor, do not use fiberglass insulation. Instead, use a continuous two-inch layer of sheet foam on the concrete under the joists.

Furnishings

Do

_____ Use a leather couch or a futon with an allergen-control encasing on the mattress, rather than upholstered pieces that can soak up body moisture and accumulate food bits, leading to mold growth and dust mite infestations. (See Part II, Dilemma 3B, "Other Rooms and Their Contents.")

_____ Keep furniture a few inches away from cool walls.

_____ Use furniture with legs long enough to allow adequate air space beneath.

Heating

Do

_____ Consistently heat all the basement rooms (60 to 65°F) in the colder months, even when you are away from home.

_____ Leave smaller spaces that lack heat (closets, cabinets) open to heated rooms, or have louvered doors installed.

Don't

_____ Let isolated spaces (rooms with closed doors, cabinets under the basement stairs, closets) go without heating.

Moisture Control

Do

_____ Determine the source of moisture condensing on surfaces. (Water can evaporate from one place and condense on a remote place where the temperature is lower.)
_____ Repair any leak.
_____ Dehumidify if the relative humidity is higher than 50%.

Recreation

Don't

_____ Exercise in a musty-smelling finished basement room.
_____ Let children play in a moldy or musty-smelling basement room or on an old basement carpet.

JEFF'S GEMS

I have seen beautifully decorated finished basement playrooms, studies, exercise rooms, bedrooms, and even home theaters infested with mold. Many of these spaces were designed for leisure activities, and people spent hours there, breathing in high concentrations of mold spores. If you exercise in a moldy basement your exposure is even greater because of your increased respiration rate.

➤ Moisture Control at the Exterior

Do

_____ Hire a professional to slope the grade (the angle of the ground) away from the foundation.

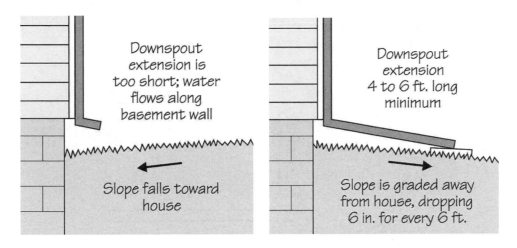

Downspout extension is too short; water flows along basement wall	Downspout extension 4 to 6 ft. long minimum
← Slope falls toward house	→ Slope is graded away from house, dropping 6 in. for every 6 ft.

Incorrect and correct grading. Around a foundation, inadequate dispersal of roof water and incorrect slope of soil or soil covering, such as concrete or asphalt, are the most common causes of below-grade dampness. *Tom Feiza, Mr. Fix-It, Inc.*

_____ Test the foundation for leaks by running water from a hose outside the area where you suspect water may be getting into the basement, but especially near where a downspout discharges rainwater. Then check the basement.

_____ To watch for water intrusion during a heavy rain

      _____ Check the basement.

      _____ Check gutters to be sure they are not overflowing.

      _____ Check downspouts to be sure they are not leaking.

CONNIE'S COMMENTS

I'm sure that Jeff is one of few people who go outside during a deluge to check the gutter system! At least he uses an umbrella to keep his camera dry. (He photographs lots of odd things, like water running down the exterior of a building and a leaking downspout.)

_____ Keep the gutter system clean and free of leaves, to avoid clogging and overflowing.

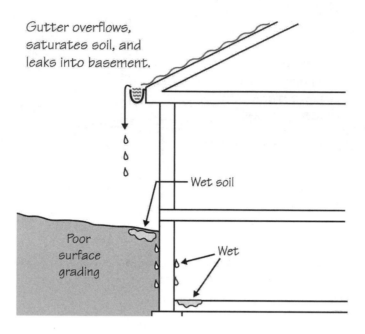

Gutter overflows, saturates soil, and leaks into basement.

Wet soil

Poor surface grading

Wet

Keep your gutters clean to reduce foundation moisture. The closer the trees, the greater the amount of leaf litter and tree debris. At houses surrounded by trees, gutters may need to be cleaned two or three times a year. Luckily, owners of a house in the middle of a field may never have to clean their gutters! *Tom Feiza, Mr. Fix-It, Inc.*

_____ Make sure people you hire to clean the gutters don't flush leaves and debris into the downspouts, clogging them.

_____ Insert the downspouts into extensions to prevent water from ponding at the foundation.

      _____ Or insert the downspouts into four-inch PVC piping that is buried just beneath the surface and exits to daylight at the edge of a landscape furrow or at a more remote, downhill location.

_____ If you don't have gutters, be sure the roof has an adequate overhang (at least eighteen inches).

_____ If the building is on the side or bottom of a hill, divert water away from the foundation with a swale (a large, shallow ditch in the soil).

_____ If all else fails, have a sub-surface deflection skirt installed around the foundation. (A sub-surface deflection skirt is an impermeable mem-

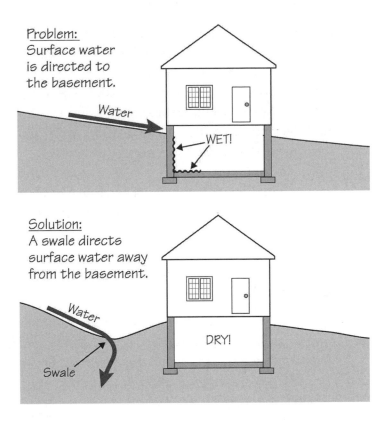

Problem:
Surface water is directed to the basement.

Water

WET!

Solution:
A swale directs surface water away from the basement.

Water

Swale

DRY!

A swale is a shallow ditch used to direct surface water away from the foundation. If you live on a hill and get basement moisture due to surface water flows, a swale may be the only solution to the problem. Installing a swale can entail an expensive excavation but will be worth the cost if it stops the water intrusion. *Tom Feiza, Mr. Fix-It, Inc.*

brane that is adhered to the foundation about 6 to 12 inches below grade, sloping away from the foundation and extending out about 30 inches.)

► For People with Allergies, Asthma, or Environmental Sensitivities

Do

_____ Send a sample of ceiling fiberglass insulation to a mold-testing lab if the insulation is exposed in a crawl space or basement or accessible above a drop ceiling in a finished basement.

_____ If the fiberglass is contaminated with moldy dust, have professionals remove it under containment. (See Part I, Dilemma 2, "Confirmation and Remediation.")
_____ After the insulation has been removed, the ceiling joists and subfloor should be HEPA vacuumed (using a vacuum with high efficiency particulate arrestance filtration) and lightly spray painted to seal in the residual dust.

_____ If paint fumes bother you, spray paint the structure with Elmer's glue and water instead of paint (approximately one to two parts water to one part glue).

CONNIE'S COMMENTS

I've heard Jeff say again and again that when people are sensitized to mold, the basement should be as clean as the rest of the house. You should be able to put a piece of jellied toast jelly side down on any basement surface, he says, and then be able to pick it up and eat it without concern. Jeff is a bit of a fanatic, but he has your best interests at heart.

_____ After HEPA vacuuming baseboard convectors in a finished basement, "super-clean" the convectors with a steam vapor machine. (See "A Finished Basement" earlier in this section.)

Don't
_____ Live in a below-grade space or in a home with a finished basement.
_____ Exercise or work in a below-grade space.

My Notes _____

_____

_____

_____

_____

_____

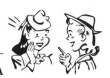

OTHER VOICES: Q & A

Q: I've set up my sewing machine in the basement, near the washer and dryer. I can spend three hours or more down there and feel fine, but when my husband is there for more than a few minutes, he coughs. He is allergic to mold. We've never had any basement water problems, and I don't see any mold. Could there be mold growth in the basement? Should I move my sewing machine upstairs?

A: Sometimes the chemicals (like detergents or enzymes) in laundry products make people cough, but if you haven't been consistently dehumidifying the basement during the warm, more humid months, there is a good chance that mildew (mold) growth is present. The mold doesn't seem to be bothering you (yet) but it may be causing your husband's symptoms.

Even if you move your sewing machine upstairs, air that may contain mold spores can still flow from your basement to the first floor. I therefore recommend that you have an IAQ professional evaluate conditions in the basement as soon as possible to give you guidance on the extent of the problem, how to get rid of the mold, and how to prevent its reoccurrence.

Until the mold is removed, your husband probably shouldn't spend much time in the basement, and the door from the basement to the first floor should remain closed.

REMINDERS

1. *Keep your crawl space clean, well-lit, and dehumidified.*
2. *Don't have a dirt floor in a basement or crawl space.*
3. *Carefully follow the manufacturer's directions when operating a steam vapor machine.*
4. *Make sure the basement remains dehumidified while you are away on your summer vacation. If necessary, ask a neighbor to monitor the relative humidity and check the dehumidifier to be sure it is working properly.*

WARNINGS

1. *Unless consistently air conditioned or dehumidified in warm, humid weather and heated in cold weather, a finished basement is prone to mildew problems.*
2. *Mold can grow in the captured dust in exposed fiberglass insulation.*

RELEVANT RESOURCES

Laboratories That Analyze Dust Samples

Aerotech Labs, Phoenix, AZ (800-651-4802, www.aerotechpk.com).
DACI Laboratory, Johns Hopkins University Asthma and Allergy Center, Baltimore, MD (800-344-3224, www.hopkinsmedicine.org/allergy/daci/index.html).
Northeast Laboratory, Winslow, ME (800-244-8378, www.nelabservices.com).

A Lab That Sells Test Kits for Mycotoxins

Envirologix, Portland, ME (866-408-4597, http://envirologix.com).

An Organization

National Institute of Occupational Safety and Health (800-311-3435, www.cdc.gov/niosh).

Products

Dehumidifier: Therma-Stor in Madison, WI (800-533-7533, www.thermastor.com).
DensShield (fiberglass-backed drywall): Available in most building supply stores.
Floor-water alarms: Available in many building supply stores.
Foil-laminated, solid sheet-form insulation: Polyisocyanurate (commonly called "polyiso"), available in most building supply stores.
HEPA vacuums: I prefer the Miele, but a number of HEPA vacuums are available online and in some specialty cleaning-equipment stores. (See www.miele.com and www.allergybuyersclub.com.)
Hygrometer: To monitor relative humidity, available online and in many hardware and building supply stores. Therma-Stor sells the "Humidity Alert," a record-

ing thermo-hygrometer (a hygrometer that also measures temperature) with an alarm (www.thermastor.com).

Mask: A two-strap, NIOSH N95 mask is available in many home supply and hardware stores. Brands and models include 3M #8210 and Gerson #1710.

Masonry Coating: Neutocrete covers dirt floors in basements and crawl spaces. Neutocrete Systems, Inc., in Holbrook, MA (888-799-9997).

MERV 7–11 filters: Available online and in many building supply stores.

Sealant: Thoroseal is a water-based Portland cement foundation sealant, manufactured by Thoro and available in most building supply stores (www.elgene.com).

Steam vapor machine: Available in some building supply stores and online. (See www.allergybuyersclub.com.) Consider a Fogacci or LadyBug machine.

Websites

www.allergybuyersclub.com for home products.
www.crawlspaces.org for information on crawl space hygiene.

B. MY ATTIC

_____ There's a musty smell in my attic.
_____ I think I see mold growth in my attic.
_____ In only one area? (This suggests that a bathroom or kitchen fan may be venting up into the attic.)
_____ I have other concerns. _____

_____

_____

_____

_____

_____

► Inspections

Do

_____ Install lighting and safe access in the attic so you can periodically check for leaks or pest infestations. (See Part II, Dilemma 3E, "Pets and Pests.")

_____ Nail 5/8- to 3/4-inch plywood down if there's no floor and you or other people plan to walk around your attic for inspections or repair.

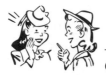

OTHER VOICES: A CASE STUDY

A contractor I knew was hired to install a vent pipe in an attic. He was concentrating on drilling a hole in the sheathing above him and lost track of where his feet were planted. The attic lacked flooring. A bathroom was located below where he stood. His feet should have been on the floor joists but instead were resting on the insulation lying on the back of the drywall of the bathroom ceiling.

He pushed against the drill and his feet plunged through the drywall ceiling, one leg on each side of a floor joist. Ouch! He let out a scream, and an instant later, so did the woman sitting on the toilet below as two legs burst through her ceiling.

➤ Moisture Control

Do

_____ In cooler climates, watch for condensation or frost on roofing nails — a sign of excess moisture — on a clear cold fall, winter, or spring night.

_____ In warmer climates, watch for condensation on attic ducts or other piping to the indoor AC unit. This is a sign of excess moisture or inadequate insulation on mechanical equipment.

_____ Check if a bathroom or kitchen exhaust fan is venting into the attic by having someone turn the fan on and off while you stand in the attic above the room in question, listening and looking for signs of air flow (moving dust or insulation).

    _____ If you can see the bathroom exhaust hose or a kitchen exhaust duct, be sure it vents to the exterior rather than terminating anywhere in the attic.

    _____ If the hose or duct doesn't vent to the exterior, hire an electrician or plumber to attach it to a vent kit that exhausts directly to the exterior.

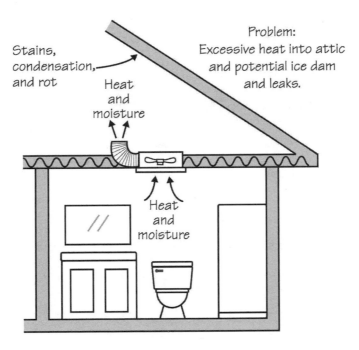

Stains, condensation, and rot

Heat and moisture

Problem: Excessive heat into attic and potential ice dam and leaks.

Heat and moisture

The most common cause of attic mold is moisture from a bathroom vented improperly into an attic. Heat from a bathroom exhaust can also cause ice dams—the buildup of ice and water at the edge of a roof. Ice dams can lead to significant roof leaks. *Tom Feiza, Mr. Fix-It, Inc.*

_____ Install a gasketed box made of sheet-foam insulation above the opening for the pull-down stairs to reduce the flow of moist house air up into the attic.

_____ Be sure an attic access panel fits tightly; consider attaching sheet-foam insulation to the back of the panel and weather-stripping along the front edges.

_____ If you want recessed lights in a room below an attic, use only fixtures that are airtight and rated "IC" (insulation contact).

_____ Have a ridge vent installed to improve attic ventilation.

      _____ Be sure the roofer cuts away the sheathing before installing the ridge vent. (Many do not take this step!)

      _____ Have continuous soffit vents installed at the same time.

_____ Make airtight any AC ducts located in the attic.

_____ Insulate AC ducts on the exterior with fiberglass.

_____ Wrap any cold water pipes present in the attic with foam-tube insulation to prevent sweating due to condensation.

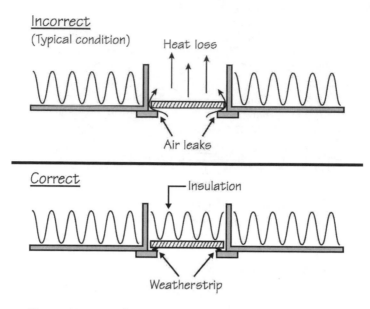

Incorrect
(Typical condition)

Heat loss

Air leaks

Correct

Insulation

Weatherstrip

The attic trapdoor can be a big air and heat loss.
It needs weatherstripping and insulation.

Another common cause of attic mold is infiltration of house moisture into the attic through gaps around attic access hatches and pull-down stairs. *Tom Feiza, Mr. Fix-It, Inc.*

JEFF'S GEMS

Mold can grow in an attic when excess moisture is present. In cooler climates, pull-down attic stairs that aren't tight-fitting and recessed lights in rooms below the attic can allow warm, moist house air to infiltrate the attic. Then moisture condenses on cooler attic surfaces. In air-conditioned buildings in warm humid climates, air from the exterior used to ventilate the attic carries moisture, which can condense on any inadequately insulated, and thus cooler, air conditioning ducts or equipment. In some very humid climates, attic ventilation may have to be reduced.

Don't

_____ Over-ventilate your attic if you live in a hot, very humid climate, such as in the Southeast.

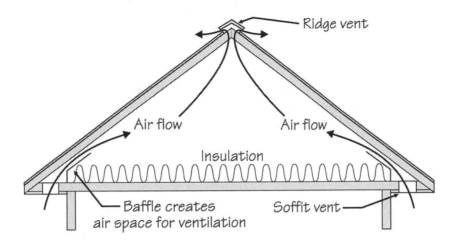

Ridge and soffit vents are the rule in new construction (but the gable-end vents in older homes can be perfectly adequate). *Tom Feiza, Mr. Fix-It, Inc.*

_____ Install circular soffit vents, which have little area for ventilation and often get clogged with paint.

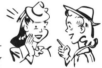

OTHER VOICES: A CASE STUDY

One homeowner asked me to help figure out why his attic felt so damp. Moisture was rising up through gaps from the rooms below, where several portable humidifiers were running. In addition, the attic did not have adequate ventilation to the exterior.

As I walked through the attic to the opposite gable end, I saw a textured black circle several feet in diameter located near the chimney on top of the foil-coated insulation. As I neared the spot, I realized that the circle consisted of thousands of carpenter ants, basking motionless in the warm, moist attic atmosphere.

To avoid being in the next Alfred Hitchcock horror film (The Ants), I quickly and quietly retreated on tiptoes to the pull-down stairs!

➤ Pipes

Don't

_____ Install water pipes in an unconditioned (neither heated nor cooled) attic if you have freezing winters.

➤ Repairs

Do

_____ Paint small areas of darkened but undamaged sheathing with an alcohol-based sealer like BIN, available in many paint, building supply, and hardware stores.

    _____ Exercise caution by following the manufacturer's directions when applying alcohol-based paint, or hire a professional to do this work.

    _____ Use supplemental ventilation (put a fan on exhaust in an attic window or gable-end vent) to remove fumes.

_____ If you are having your roof repaired or the roofing replaced, be sure the exposed work area can be protected should it rain (especially if there is plank sheathing).

_____ Temporarily cover with plastic any goods stored in the attic when a new roof is being installed.

_____ Any sections of attic sheathing that are delaminated or decayed due to moisture and fungal growth should be replaced.

Don't

_____ Postpone repairing roof leaks.

➤ Storage

Don't

_____ Use an attic for storage unless there is securely attached plywood or a plank floor in the trafficked areas.

➤ For People with Allergies, Asthma, or Environmental Sensitivities

Do

_____ When going up into a dusty attic, wear a NIOSH (National Institute of Occupational Safety and Health) N95 mask, available in most hardware and building supply stores.

_____ Change your clothes after being in a dusty attic.

_____ Have exposed attic insulation that is full of dead insects or rodent litter removed under containment. (See Part I, Dilemma 1A, "My Basement.")

    _____ The floor and attic structure should then be HEPA vacuumed (using a vacuum cleaner with high efficiency particulate arrestance filtration) and lightly paint sealed to contain potentially allergenic dust before the insulation is replaced.

    _____ If paint smells bother you, you can use a solution of Elmer's glue and water (approximately one to two parts water to one part glue).

    _____ To prevent the spread of contaminated dust indoors, see if workers can safely enter and exit the attic via a ladder placed up against a temporary wall hole that opens directly to the exterior.

Don't

_____ Use items covered with attic dust without HEPA vacuuming them first.

My Notes _____

_____

_____

_____

_____

_____

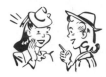

OTHER VOICES: Q & A

Q: Because the air in our house was so dry, we just added a humidifier to the hot-air heating system located in our basement. Now I'm noticing mold in the attic for the first time. Could the humidifier be causing mold to grow?

A: You bet. Be sure there is adequate ventilation in the attic space to the outside, and that there are no openings through which your now moister house air can leak into the attic. In addition, if there are any supply ducts in the attic, check for gaps or air leaks in the ductwork that could introduce more moisture into the attic space. Monitor the home's relative humidity (RH) with a hygrometer, and don't let the RH get over 40%. On very cold winter days (temperature below 20°F), even 35% may be excessive.

Q: We live in an old Victorian, and half of our attic is finished off into a guest bedroom with a built-in bureau along one wall. I keep sheets and blankets in that bureau, and when I take the bedding out of a drawer it smells musty. When my daughter visits me, she sleeps in that room. She says the smell of the sheets makes her cough, so I have to wash the sheets again before I make the bed for her. Is there any way to prevent the bedding from smelling like this?

A: When those bureau drawers are closed they may extend back into the unfinished attic eaves. Pull out a drawer and look behind it. Can you see the sheathing or insulation? If so, the bedding is open to hundred-year-old dust that may contain pest droppings, rodent nesting materials, dead flies, and mold spores (which, even if dead, can be irritating to those who are sensitized). No wonder the sheets smell!

You can hire a carpenter to build an enclosure for the back and sides of the bureau, isolating the drawers from the attic eaves. Or you could stop using the bureau and seal the edges of the drawers with adhesive-backed, insulating foam strips, because in certain weather conditions air can flow from the attic eaves into the room around the edges of the drawers, even when they are closed.

JEFF'S GEMS

I'm more worried about mold in a basement than in an attic. Mold spores are carried on air currents, and hot air rises. In a colder climate, air moves in a heated building from bottom to top — from the basement to the rooms above and then to the attic. In a hot, humid climate, the attic is heated by the sun during the day, so attic air tends to be hotter than the air outside and flows upward to the exterior of the building rather than down to the rooms below.

Mold spores in an attic don't tend to spread to the rooms below unless there is mechanical equipment for an air conveyance system (hot-air heat, central air conditioning) in the attic. Then spores can find their way into the system through gaps in the ducts and be circulated throughout the building. If mold growth in a basement is disturbed, however, spores and other byproducts of mold growth can easily be carried on air flowing up into the habitable rooms above.

REMINDERS

1. *Never exhaust bathrooms or dryers up into the attic.*
2. *Install lighting and safe access so you can inspect conditions in the attic.*
3. *Check with a ventilation professional or roofer in your area to be sure that openings in ridge and soffit vents are not blocked and are of sufficient size for their purpose.*

WARNINGS

1. *In a cold climate, water dripping from or ice forming on nail heads in the attic is a sign of excess moisture.*
2. *In a hot and humid climate, condensation on the surfaces of mechanical equipment in an attic may be a sign of inadequate AC duct insulation or excess attic ventilation.*

An Organization

National Institute of Occupational Safety and Health (800-311-3435, www.cdc.gov/niosh).

Products

BIN: An alcohol-based stain sealer available in many building supply and hardware stores.

Hygrometer: Available in many building supply and hardware stores, this device measures the relative humidity (RH). Therma-Stor sells a recording thermo-hygrometer (a hygrometer that also measures temperature) with an alarm (www.thermastor.com).

NIOSH N95 mask: Available in many hardware and building supply stores. Brands and models include 3M #8210 and Gerson #1710.

C. THE ROOMS IN BETWEEN

———— There are musty smells in certain rooms.
    In which rooms? ————————————————————

———— I can see mildew on walls.
    In which rooms? ————————————————————

———— I can see mildew on ceilings or behind pictures.
    In which rooms? ————————————————————

———— I found a mushroom inside my house.
    Where? ————————————————————————

———— I have other concerns. ————————————————

————————————————————————————————————

————————————————————————————————————

———————————————————————————————

JEFF'S GEMS

Some vinyl products such as window trim or even computer components can smell musty due to chemical off-gassing. (See Part II, Dilemma 3B, "Other

Rooms and Their Contents.") Also, some mold growth smells musty and other mold growth can be odorless. So if a room has a musty smell, it doesn't mean that extensive mold growth is present. By the same token, a room that has no mold odor can contain a lot of mildew.

CONNIE'S COMMENTS

Not very comforting, is he? Still, one way to find out if there's mildew in your home is to look for it, whether you detect a musty smell or not.

➤ Musty Odors

Do

_____ Sniff the window trim and other vinyl materials in the room where there is an odor.

　　　_____ If you think something vinyl smells musty, remove it from the room if possible to see if the smell goes away.

　　　_____ If the object cannot be removed, cover it with aluminum foil to see if the musty smell diminishes.

_____ Put a box fan on exhaust in a window and close the other doors and windows in the room.

JEFF'S GEMS

When you set up negative pressure in a room with a box fan, air will flow from the wall and ceiling cavities into the room through construction gaps, electric outlets, light fixtures, and other openings. The strongest smell will emanate from those openings nearest the odor source — perhaps microbial growth in the HVAC (heating, ventilation, and air conditioning) system or mold growth or a pest infestation inside a wall or ceiling cavity. (Refer to Part I, Dilemma 2, "Confirmation and Remediation," and Part II, Dilemma 3E, "Pets and Pests.")

_____ Sniff around the heat or air conditioning registers and grilles for odor.

    _____ If they smell, hire an IAQ professional or an HVAC technician to investigate. (See Part I, Dilemma 1F, "Heating and Cooling Systems.")

_____ If you don't detect an odor around the registers and grilles, cover them with foil and removable painters' tape so you can sniff for other odor sources.

    _____ Cautiously sniff around electric outlets, light fixtures, and other openings in the ceiling or walls. Sniff every gap or crack, even those as small as a gap between a piece of wood trim and a wall.

    _____ If you find a smelly opening, hire a professional to open up that area of the wall or ceiling — either under containment (see Part I, Dilemma 1A, "My Basement"), or from the outside if possible — to locate the mold growth (though a pest infestation may be the culprit).

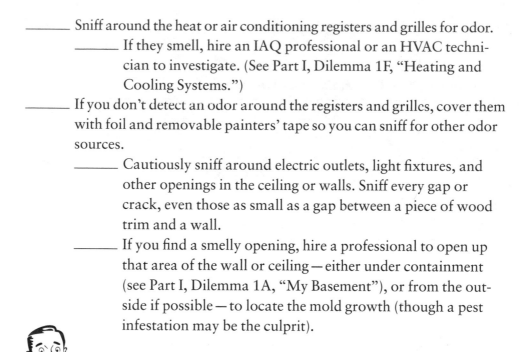

JEFF'S GEMS

A kitchen, bathroom, laundry area, and even a room that contains a hot tub or pool can be prone to mildew growth because of the presence of moisture. It's not unusual to see mold under a kitchen sink where a pipe has leaked or on the ceiling in a bathroom, near the tub/shower enclosure. And I've seen the underside of hot-tub and pool covers covered with mold. We can do without in-home laundries, pools, and hot tubs, though they are wonderful conveniences and luxuries, but we have to have a place to cook meals, go to the bathroom, and bathe. You can exercise some simple precautions, however, that will help you avoid mold problems in these rooms.

► Rooms with Water

Bathrooms

Do

_____ Check the escutcheon plate on the tub overflow. If loose, it is leaking and should be fixed.

_____ Gently tap wall tiles and floor tiles with the handle of a screw-driver at the edge of the tub and around valves to see if any tiles are loose.

      _____ Have loose tiles repaired.

      _____ Have loose or missing grout replaced.

_____ Keep the shower curtain inside the tub or the shower doors closed when showering.

_____ If you have a shower curtain for your bathtub, use splash guards at the tub ends.

_____ Cover a window in a shower enclosure with its own shower curtain.

      _____ Such windows should be made of safety glass.

_____ Keep shower doors clean, including the door tracks.

_____ Check outside a tub enclosure for leaks when someone is showering.

_____ Dry yourself off before stepping out of a shower or tub enclosure.

_____ After showering, reduce moisture in the room.

      _____ Keep the bathroom door open and air out the room with an open window or exhaust fan.

      _____ Operate a small, oscillating wall-mounted table-top or floor-standing fan to mix the air and speed evaporation. (Always plug electrical equipment in a bathroom into a GFI — ground fault interrupt — outlet.)

      _____ If these steps don't prevent mold from growing on the walls and ceiling and you live in a cold climate, consider improving wall and/or ceiling insulation.

_____ Using a mirror and bright flashlight, check under the sink periodically for leaks.

      _____ If there is a leak, have it repaired as soon as possible.

_____ If your toilet is leaking, have it repaired.

JEFF'S GEMS

One man found a mushroom growing out of the wood floor next to his toilet. He figured the problem was solved when he picked the mushroom. Mush-rooms can be signs of extensive, concealed fungal growth, however, and the *kind of fungus that produces mushrooms rots wood. If you find a mushroom growing in your home, call a contractor or an experienced home inspector — a member of the American Society of Home Inspectors (www.ashi.org) — to determine the cause of the problem and assess the need for repairs.*

Don't

_____ Fill a bathtub above the bottom of the overflow (escutcheon) plate.

_____ Let wet towels sit in clumps on the bathroom floor.

_____ Hang-dry clothes or towels in a bathroom if you are battling mold growth in the room.

_____ Use corn-starch body powder. Unlike talc body powder, it is biodegradable.

_____ Let bathroom floor mats get saturated with water.

_____ Have a wall-to-wall carpet in a bathroom.

JEFF'S GEMS

When I see wall-to-wall carpeting in bathrooms, kitchens, entranceways, laundry areas, and porches open to the weather, I know I'm looking at a potential mold problem.

Kitchens

Do

_____ Check the floor in front of your dishwasher for a hump or discoloration that might be due to a leak.

_____ Rinse the food from dishes before putting them in the dishwasher.

_____ Check under the sink with a mirror and flashlight for leaks from hoses and valves.

      _____ If there is a leak, have it repaired as soon as possible.

_____ Dry between the sink and backsplash if water accumulates in that area when you use the sink.

_____ If you have a water line for ice or cold water in the refrigerator

_____ Check the line at the back for leaks.

_____ Check the floor in front of the appliance for stains or floor swelling.

_____ Clean the inside of your refrigerator twice a year with a suitable household cleaner.

_____ Put two or three tablespoons of salt in a removable plastic (not metal) refrigerator drip tray to deter mold, yeast, and bacterial growth. (If you don't know whether your refrigerator has a removable drip tray, check the manufacturer's instruction booklet.)

_____ Use a 36-inch crevice tool (see www.vacuumstore.com), attached to a HEPA vacuum, to

_____ Keep the refrigerator coils dust-free.

_____ Clean around and below the refrigerator once or twice a year.

_____ Keep the refrigerator door open if you unplug the appliance, for example, when you are moving. (Even if the appliance is empty, there are still invisible bits of food on the walls and in the drawers.)

_____ Use a stove exhaust fan vented to the exterior when cooking.

Don't

_____ Leave your dishwasher door closed if the machine is full of dirty dishes and you plan to be away from the house for several days.

_____ Let moldy food remain in your refrigerator or garbage can.

_____ Keep your garbage around in the house for more than one day.

_____ Have wall-to-wall carpet in the kitchen.

Laundry Areas

Do

_____ Check your washing machine periodically for leaks, using a mirror and flashlight if necessary.

_____ Shut off the water supply valves when the washing machine is not in use, particularly when you will be away from the house for more than a few days.

_____ Use water hoses that are stainless-steel covered.

_____ Install a drain and waterproof containment tray under a washing machine if it's not located in the basement.

_____ If the washing-machine drain is part of the plumbing system, keep the trap filled with water to prevent sewer gas from exiting the pipe.

_____ Have a floor water alarm near your washing machine.

   _____ If you have a central alarm system, install a floor water alarm that connects to that system.

_____ Remove lint that has accumulated around the base of the washing-machine agitator or in the bleach container.

_____ To reduce lint in house dust, clean the clogged screen outdoors. Buy a spare screen so you won't have to go outdoors between loads.

_____ To facilitate drying, keep the washing-machine door open when the machine is not in use.

_____ In a front-loading washing machine, clean the gaskets inside and out every few weeks.

_____ Vent a dryer to the exterior, rather than into the laundry area, attic, basement, garage, crawl space, or under a deck.

_____ Wherever possible, use solid metal vent piping with few elbows rather than flexible hose for your dryer exhaust.

_____ Check periodically to see that air is exiting the vent kit; a clogged hose can be a fire hazard and must be cleaned.

_____ Check behind the dryer periodically (use a mirror and flashlight) to be certain that the dryer hose is connected and not kinked.

Don't

_____ Use a line trap (a plastic tub that collects dryer moisture and lint indoors).

_____ Use a dryer-hose damper valve that allows you the option of diverting dryer exhaust to the interior.

_____ Have a distance of more than 20 to 25 feet between the dryer and the wall through which it exhausts. (Check the manufacturer's recommendation.)

_____ Place your washing machine on a rug or wall-to-wall carpet.

Pools and Hot Tubs Indoors

Do

_____ Periodically disinfect the bottom side of an indoor hot tub or pool cover.

_____ Keep the hot tub or pool cover as dust-free as possible.

► Rooms without Water

Carpets and Rugs

Do

_____ If you spill liquid on one small area of carpet, blot up the liquid as quickly as possible and use a fan to hasten drying.

_____ Place a small area rug that can be washed or replaced in front of doors leading to the exterior.

Don't

_____ Have carpeting in a closet with cold exterior walls (walls on the perimeter of the building).

_____ Wet the carpeting under and around potted plants.

_____ Place a plastic runner or carpet-protector over damp carpeting.

Furnishings and Possessions

Do

_____ Use a bright flashlight, held almost parallel to surfaces, to look for mildew growth (a thin layer of fuzz or white, pale blue-green, or yellow round or oval spots) on the legs, sides, and backs of furniture.

_____ Use a mirror as well as flashlight to look at the bottoms of furniture.

_____ Keep plant pots on moisture-proof barriers.

_____ Put a towel over your pillow if you go to bed with damp hair.

_____ Store shoes on a rack above a closet floor, especially if the closet is unheated and has an exterior wall.

Don't

_____ Keep musty-smelling sofas, cushions, pillows, or mattresses.

_____ Keep thick clothing that still smells musty after being washed or dry-cleaned.

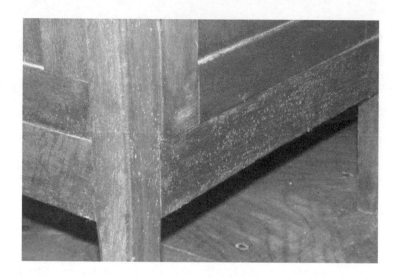

This desk was probably stored in a basement before it was placed in a bedroom. The white mold colonies only became visible because the camera flash illuminated them from an angle. *May Indoor Air Investigations LLC*

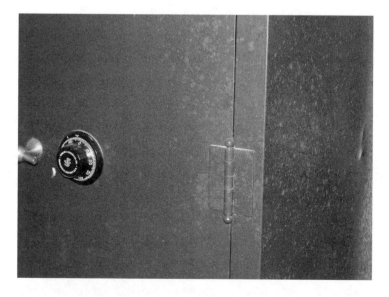

This safe was in a basement that was not dehumidified. Mold grew on the dust that had settled on the sides. *May Indoor Air Investigations LLC*

_____ Acquire musty-smelling, upholstered furniture.

_____ Store upholstered furniture in a cool, damp basement or garage.

CONNIE'S COMMENTS

After my parents died, my brother, sister, and I split up their furniture. I got their long wooden black bench with a back stenciled with gold flowers. I put the bench in the hallway outside our bedroom. Jeff coughed whenever he walked by the bench. He started complaining that the bench smelled musty and was making him feel sick — an assertion I looked on with some suspicion, I must admit. I thought perhaps he just didn't like the bench. When he found extensive mildew growth on the bottom of it, I felt bad! We took the bench outside where I cleaned off the mold with denatured alcohol and then covered the underside with clear shellac to seal in any residual spores. After that, the bench was no longer a problem for Jeff. (Refer to Part I, Dilemma 2B, "Cleaning It Up Myself.")

_____ Over-humidify your home for your plants' sake (unless you want to grow mold!).

_____ Let dead leaves that drop from your plant accumulate on the soil.

_____ Keep your Christmas tree too long. (It can get moldy.)

_____ Regularly go to bed with wet hair, dampening the pillow.

_____ Store clothing flush against cold exterior walls in closets.

_____ Place shoes directly on the floor if there's concrete under the carpet.

OTHER VOICES: Q & A

Q: We stayed a few days in my cousin's house, and when we came home, our clothes smelled musty. My cousin doesn't believe that mold can be transported on clothing, but I think he's wrong. Could we have carried a mold problem back to our own house?

A: Mold odors can be pervasive, and clothing can adsorb such smells, collecting the smells on the surfaces of the fibers. Despite the presence of a moldy odor in clothing, however, there might not be any spores present. On the other hand, if mold was disturbed when you were nearby, your clothing may contain spores as well as mold-eating mites. Still, this is not that different from picking up spores on your clothing as you walk among moldy leaves in your yard on a fall day. Have the clothing washed or dry-cleaned, and the odor as well as any mold spores should be eliminated.

Heating in Cold Climates

Do
_____ Keep a closet with exterior walls and mildew problems warm by leaving the door open, having a louvered door, or adding a heater designed for closets (www.omega.com).
_____ Keep rooms you inhabit consistently heated to at least 60°F in winter, and rooms over cold crawl spaces and garages a few degrees warmer.
_____ In rooms you rarely enter (and therefore keep cooler in the winter), keep doors closed and airtight with gaskets to prevent warm, moist air from entering.

Don't
_____ Keep the heat below 55°F in a colder climate if you tend to have mold problems.

Walls and Doors

Do
_____ Use a bright flashlight, held almost parallel to the surface, to inspect for fuzzy mold colonies (white, pale blue-green, or yellow round or oval spots) on walls and doors, especially along the bottom few feet near the floor and in closets with an exterior wall.
_____ Look carefully around windows and skylights for water stains.
_____ If a window or skylight is leaking, have it repaired.

_____ Lift up a corner of a wall-to-wall carpet and check the carpet tack-strip for rusty nails and stained or decayed wood: signs of moisture problems.

      _____ Hire a professional to figure out the moisture source and make necessary repairs.

_____ In air-conditioned rooms in hot and humid climates, check behind pictures for mold growth on the wall or back of the picture.

JEFF'S GEMS

If the air pressure indoors is less than the air pressure outdoors, outdoor air will infiltrate the wall of a building. In hot, humid climates, warm, moist outside air may then enter wall cavities. In air-conditioned spaces, this moisture will condense on the cooler backs of the drywall. Moisture can migrate through the drywall and fuel mold growth behind vinyl wallpaper, which traps the moisture. If the drywall is coated on the finished side with porous wallpaper or paint, moisture can travel to the wall surface facing the room. If that moisture can evaporate into the drier room air, mold will not grow on the wall surface. If evaporation is minimized, however, by a picture hanging on the wall, mold may grow on the surface behind the picture as well as on the back of the picture itself.

_____ Refer to Part I, Dilemmas 2B and 2C, "Cleaning It Up Myself" and "Hiring Professionals to Remediate."

► Soot, Not Mold

Do

_____ If there are black strips and dots on your walls, rub a black area with a clean, white paper towel until some of the black is on the towel. Wearing protective gloves and eye protection, add a few drops of bleach to the towel. If the marks don't disappear, they are probably soot.

JEFF'S GEMS

Jar candles as well as poorly tuned heating equipment can produce soot, which can cause thousands of dollars of cosmetic damage to walls and ceilings, but which is not mold. Soot can appear as black spots about the size of a screw head at each drywall fastener, stripes at studs on walls or rafters in ceilings, dark ceiling spots directly above wall or ceiling light fixtures, and flame-like patterns above baseboard convectors.

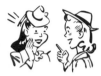

OTHER VOICES: A CASE STUDY

A woman with two young children saw black stain patterns on the ceilings in her dining room and kitchen. She was worried the spots might be mold and could affect her children's health, so she sent a sample of the black stain to a lab, which identified the material as "toxic black mold." The lab technician advised the woman to move immediately out of her house. She and her children were living in a trailer parked in her driveway when she called me.

The stains turned out to be soot and not mold. The woman had her home repainted and stopped burning jar candles, and the soot never returned. Both her children had asthma. Soot particles aren't healthy to breathe, particularly for those who have respiratory problems. Soot particles, which are extremely small, can remain airborne for long periods of time, can carry allergenic substances, and can be inhaled deeply into the lung.

► **For People with Allergies, Asthma, or Environmental Sensitivities**

Do

_____ Discard musty-smelling or moldy-covered books or other paper goods, or store them in airtight plastic bins.

_____ Have rugs temporarily removed from a room in which you experience health symptoms.

_____ If you cough, sneeze, or wheeze in a wall-to-wall carpeted area,

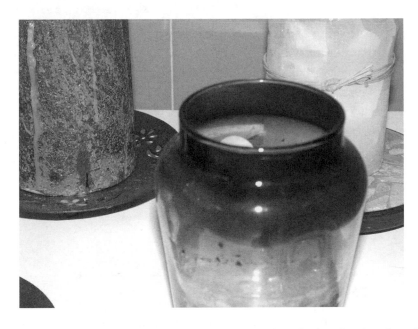

The black band at the rim and upper portion of the jar is all soot, deposited on the glass from the candle flame. This deposit represents only a small part of the soot that goes into the air from such candles. *May Indoor Air Investigations LLC*

temporarily cover the carpeting with an adhesive-backed carpet protector (www.pro-tect.com).

_____ Do not do this if the carpet is damp. (See Part 1, Dilemma 1D, "Floods and Leaks.")

_____ Wear a respirator or a mask with a NIOSH (National Institute of Occupational Safety and Health) rating of N95 if you have to enter a musty-smelling or moldy area, or if potentially moldy materials are being moved.

_____ Have containment set up if any moldy materials are being disturbed. (See Part I, Dilemma 1A, "My Basement," and Part I, Dilemma 2, "Confirmation and Remediation.")

Don't

_____ Spend prolonged time in a musty-smelling or visibly moldy space.

_____ Touch or disturb objects that smell musty or contain visible mildew, including books.

_____ Remain in a space in which other people are handling moldy goods.

_____ Use a laundry detergent that contains enzymes, because some are similar in structure to mold enzymes and can cause allergic sensitization.

My Notes _____

_____

_____

_____

_____

REMINDERS

1. *Many antiques have at some time been stored in a damp space and therefore contain mildew growth.*
2. *Be sure your shower doors are watertight.*
3. *Soot is not mold.*

WARNINGS

1. *Over-humidifying a space can lead to mold growth, especially on cooler surfaces.*
2. *Venting a dryer indoors adds excess moisture and biodegradable lint to the interior of your home.*
3. *Mushrooms indoors indicate the presence of wood-degrading fungi and a long-term problem with moisture.*

RELEVANT RESOURCES

An Organization

American Society of Home Inspectors, Des Plaines, IL (800-743-2744, www.ashi.org).

Products

Adhesive-backed carpet protector: Pro-Tect (www.pro-tect.com).

Floor water alarm: Available in building supply stores and online
  (www.gizmode.com/).

Heaters for closets: www.omega.com.

NIOSH N95 mask, available in many hardware and building supply stores. Brands
  include 3M #8210 and Gerson #1710.

Vacuum attachment to clean refrigerator coil (a 36-inch crevice tool): Available in
  some vacuum supply stores and online. Search for "vacuum" and "crevice
  tool" (and see www.midamericavacuum.com or www.vacuumstore.com).

D. FLOODS AND LEAKS

_____ I had a flood in my basement.

_____ A burst pipe led to staining on a ceiling or wall.

_____ My roof leaked and caused cosmetic damage in rooms below.

_____ There's a musty smell or mold growth where a leak or flood
  occurred. (See Part I, Dilemma 1C, "The Rooms In Between.")

_____ I have other concerns. _____

_____

_____

➤ Floods

Do

_____ Keep careful written and photographic records of a flood and the
  damage caused by the flooding.
  When did the flood start? _____
  Where did the flood happen? _____
  When was the problem reported and to whom? _____
  What actions were taken, by whom, and when? _____

_____

_____ Have someone monitor your home for floods when you are away on
  vacation.

_____ Refer to Part I, Dilemma 1F, "Heating and Cooling Systems," for tips about avoiding leaks and flooding caused by hot-water heaters.

_____ Keep any basement that has been flooded isolated from habitable spaces during the drying out process.

    _____ Close and cover with plastic all doors leading upstairs.

    _____ Seal pipe openings with tape or insulation.

    _____ Open the basement windows.

    _____ Remove soggy objects and materials through an opening with direct access to the exterior rather than through the house.

_____ Call professionals to clean and dry wall-to-wall carpeting that has been flooded with clean water. (Carpeting flooded with black water, which is water tainted by human waste, should be discarded.)

_____ Have flooded area rugs professionally cleaned and dried off-site if possible.

_____ Discard carpeting, rugs, and carpet pads that have become wet even once if they smell or cannot be dried out completely within 24 to 48 hours.

_____ Dry out or replace walls affected by flooding, particularly if saturated.

_____ Discard wet insulation.

_____ Have professionally cleaned and disinfected any hot-air furnace or air conditioning system that was under clean water.

_____ Consult your health department and a heating contractor for advice about remediation after a fire or flood.

Black Water (water tainted by human waste)

Do

_____ Consider replacing any hot-air furnace or air conditioning system that was contaminated by black water.

_____ Replace anything fleecy, cushioned, or made of fibrous materials (mattresses, couch cushioning, carpeting, and carpet pad) that was wet by black water.

_____ Contact a restoration professional to clean up a sewer backup in the basement.

Don't

_____ Keep sofas and mattresses that have been soaked with black water.

_____ Operate a fan in a flooded, moldy basement unless you wear respiratory protection and keep the basement isolated from the rest of the house.

_____ Keep any carpeting or carpet pad that was dampened or flooded with black water.

➤ Insurance

Do

_____ Check your insurance policy to see if it covers damage from mold growth due to a leak or flood.

     _____ Consider paying for a mold rider if your insurance policy excludes mold.

_____ Keep in touch with your insurance company to be sure a water problem is dealt with quickly, efficiently, and professionally.

Don't

_____ Postpone drying out an area affected by a leak or flood because you are waiting to hear from your insurance company.

_____ Make an insurance claim for mold remediation unless the claim is for a covered loss such as a pipe leak.

➤ Leaks

Do

_____ Keep careful written and photographic records of any leak-associated damage.

When did the leak start? _____

Where was the leak located? _____

How extensive does the leak appear to be? _____

When was problem reported and to whom? _____

What actions were taken, by whom, and when? _____

_____

_____

_____ Have someone monitor your home for leaks while you are away on vacation.

JEFF'S GEMS

Use a mirror and a bright flashlight when searching for the extent of damage caused by a leak. Start at the leak level and work your way down and across to search for all areas that might have been impacted. Don't forget to look behind furniture or file cabinets that are up against exterior walls and to check the basement. For substantial leaks, have a home inspector or a building consultant test the area with a moisture meter or scan the area with a thermal imaging (infrared) camera to figure out the extent of the problem.

_____ Circle a water stain lightly and accurately at the edges with chalk or a pencil. If the staining then spreads beyond your line, the leak that caused the stain is probably ongoing.

_____ Periodically scrutinize the ceilings located under the roof, the inside of perimeter walls, under windows, and in the basement during a heavy rain to see if rainwater is getting into the building.

    _____ If there are signs that rainwater is seeping into the building, hire someone to find the cause and have the problem repaired.

_____ Do all you can to dry up moisture from a leak as quickly as possible.

_____ Apply a stain sealant such as BIN, available in many paint, building supply, and hardware stores, to a leak stain prior to repainting the area.

    _____ Be sure the leak has been repaired and the area is dry before you paint the stain.

_____ If you live in a condominium, promptly notify maintenance personnel and/or your condo association of any leaks into or in your unit.

Don't
_____ Postpone repairing or replacing your roofing.

► For People with Allergies, Asthma, or Environmental Sensitivities

Do

_____ If paint smells bother you and you are repainting a stained area on a wall or ceiling, test-apply a primer/sealer paint like BIN and then the paint you plan to use on a piece of wood outside. Wait to see if the dried paint film bothers you.

My Notes _____

_____

_____

_____

_____

_____

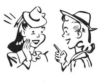

OTHER VOICES: A CASE STUDY

One home was extensively renovated after a major flood occurred on the first floor, but the original subfloor and maple floor, which had been saturated, were left in place. Mold grew between the two layers of wood, and then mold-eating mites moved in. Eventually the mold and mites died, but for twelve years, when the owners walked on the wall-to-wall carpeting, they compressed the air trapped under the warped maple flooring. Mold and mite allergens were then blown out through gaps between the subfloor boards in the basement ceiling below. One of the owners was highly allergic to the dust and developed asthma after spending many weekend hours in his basement shop.

REMINDERS

1. *Contact your insurance company immediately after a flood.*
2. *Trained professionals should clean up after a major flood.*
3. *Professionals* must *handle the cleanup of major leakage or flooding from black water.*

WARNINGS

1. *If mold is growing on a wall or ceiling where a leak occurred, there is probably mold growth on the back of the drywall as well as in any dust in fibrous insulation.*
2. *If you postpone drying an area affected by a leak or flood, you may very well end up with a mold problem or even a mold disaster.*

RELEVANT RESOURCES

Organizations

American Society of Home Inspectors, Des Plaines, IL (800-743-2744, www.ashi.org).

Munters Corporation has offices nationwide (www.muntersamerica.com) and specializes in emergency flood remediation (dehumidifying, drying).

Northeast Document Conservation Center, Andover, MA (978-470-1010, www.nedcc.org) works to recover documents damaged by flooding.

Products

BIN, an alcohol-based sealer: Available in many paint, building supply, and hardware stores.

Floor water alarm: Available in many building supply stores and online (www.gizmode.com/).

Hygrometer that measures temperature and has an alarm and recording capacity: A thermo-hygrometer, available through Therma-Stor (www.thermastor.com).

Publications

"Cleaning Up Your House after a Flood," Canadian Mortgage and Housing Corporation (613-748-2367).

"Flood Cleanup: Avoiding Indoor Air Quality Problems," EPA 402-F-93-005, August 1993 (www.epa.gov/iaq or IAQ INFO, PO Box 37133, Washington, DC 20013-7133, 800-438-4318).

"Rebuilding Flood-Damaged Homes," Alliance for Healthy Homes, March 15,

2007 (www.afhh.org/res/res＿pubs/shrfdh.pdf or PO Box 75941, Washington, DC 20013).

Standard and Reference Guide for Professional Water Damage Restoration S500–94. Vancouver, Washington Institute of Inspection, Cleaning, and Restoration Certification, 1995.

A Website

www.moldupdate.com offers general information on mold litigation and insurance issues.

E. THE GARAGE

_____ I can see mold
      _____ On walls.
      _____ On the ceiling.
      _____ On stored goods.
      _____ On the inside of the overhead door.
_____ There's a musty smell.
_____ I have other concerns. _____
_____
_____

Do
_____ If there's a musty smell
      _____ Look for black spots of mildew on the lower few feet of garage doors.
      _____ Look for less visible spots of mildew growth (fuzzy white, light yellow, or pale-green oval spots) on walls, stored items, and shelving by holding a bright flashlight almost parallel to surfaces.
      _____ Follow tips for cleaning in Part I, Dilemma 2, "Confirmation and Remediation."
_____ Use rolling metal or plastic shelves for storage.
_____ Remove as much snow from your car as you can before driving it into the garage.
_____ Keep the garage free of moldy leaves.

_____ Increase the ventilation on dry days.

_____ Repair any roof leaks.

_____ Use a dehumidifier as a last resort but only if your garage is fairly airtight and moisture cannot be reduced by other means.

_____ Clean mold from the back of the garage door and paint the surface to seal it.

        _____ Wearing protective gloves and eye protection, use a diluted bleach solution (one part bleach to ten parts water) or a household cleaner suited for the purpose; follow manufacturer's directions.

OTHER VOICE: A CASE STUDY

During a visit to some friends I hadn't seen for years, I noticed a streak of green moss and a long, damp-looking vertical stain on the brick veneer at the external corner where the meticulously maintained two-story house met the attached single-story garage. It appeared as if the garage roof had a leak. When I walked into the garage I could see patches of black mold on the drywall. The patches mirrored the water stain outside. The roof leak had to be repaired and the moldy drywall, as well as the moldy, damp insulation, had to be removed and replaced.

CONNIE'S COMMENTS

I was with him. He walked into the garage to see if he could find mold before he even said hello to his friends!

Don't

_____ Have drywall touching the concrete floor.

_____ Vent a dryer into the garage.

_____ Store cardboard boxes directly on the concrete floor or up against the concrete walls.

_____ Use wooden shelves in contact with the floor or walls to store personal goods.

My Notes _____

_____

_____

_____

_____

_____

_____

OTHER VOICES: Q & A

Q: Our driveway slopes steeply toward the house. When it rains hard, water gets into the garage and from there into the adjacent basement space. How can we solve this problem?

A: See if drainage can be installed at the bottom of the driveway in front of the garage. If this is not possible, you may want to consider abandoning the garage and converting it into basement space by building a waterproof foundation wall and filling in the driveway to create a parking area.

REMINDER

Maintain your garage roof with the same care as the roof over the rest of your house.

WARNING

Drywall touching a cool or damp concrete floor can acquire mildew growth.

F. HEATING AND COOLING SYSTEMS

_____ I can smell mold when the heating or air conditioning (AC) system is on.
_____ I or someone in my family tends to get sick more often when the
heating or air conditioning system is on.
_____ I have other concerns. _____
_____
_____

Questions to Answer

1. How is your heat supplied — by forced air in ducts, by hot water in radiators or baseboard convectors, or by steam in radiators? _____
2. Where is your boiler or furnace? _____
   (A boiler heats water for radiators and baseboard convectors or steam for radiators. A furnace heats air and can contain a cooling coil for summer AC use.)
3. Do you have a hydro-air system?
   (A hydro-air system has a boiler to heat water that is piped to two or more remote air-handling units, or AHUs, with heating coils.)
4. If you have a heat pump, where is the indoor unit located? _____
   (A heat pump is a split system with an indoor unit and an outdoor unit. The blower and heat exchange coil, together called the air-handling unit, are indoors, and the compressor is outdoors.)
5. Do you have an air conveyance system?
   (An air conveyance system uses air, one or more blowers, and ducts to deliver warm or cool air.)
   Do you have metal or flexible ducts? _____
   If metal, are they insulated on the inside? _____
   Do you have fiberglass ducts covered with aluminum foil (duct board)? ___
   Are there ducts in the attic? _____
   As far as you know, do any ducts run through concrete, such as a concrete slab? _____
   Do you have any returns that are panned bays (spaces between joists, lined at the bottom with sheet metal or drywall)? _____
   Do you know the type and location of the filter? _____

6. If you have air conditioning, is it:
   A central system? _____
   A newer, mini-split system? _____
   (A mini-split system has one or more indoor, wall-mounted AC units and an outdoor compressor.)
   A window or through-wall AC? _____
   A portable AC? _____
7. Do you have humidification? _____
   If so, is it a central system? _____ What kind? _____
   Or is it a portable unit? _____ Where do you use it and how often? _____
8. Do you have dehumidification? _____
   If so, it is a central system? _____ What kind? _____
   Or is it a portable dehumidifier? _____ What kind? _____
   Where do you use it and how often? _____

JEFF'S GEMS

Mold in a mechanical system is a common source of building odors and indoor air quality problems. Yet when I ask clients about their heating or cooling system, more often than not I am greeted with blank stares. The only component of the system people are often familiar with is the thermostat, which is why I see so many air quality problems in homes.

The questions above aren't all directly connected to indoor air quality, but please take some time to try to answer them nonetheless. Have a knowledgeable friend, HVAC (heating, ventilation, and air conditioning) technician, or an ASHI (American Society of Home Inspectors) professional explain the basic components of your heating or cooling system to you. At the end, you should know what type of system you have, where the sources of heating and cooling are located, and where to find your filters and access panels, among other practical details of the workings of the system. Then you can ask questions relevant to your indoor air quality concerns, as well as be more knowledgeable when your mechanical system develops mold and other problems.

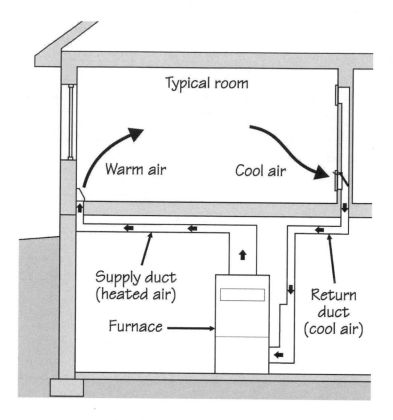

The air conveyance system consists of the furnace itself and the return and supply ducts. Air that is drawn by the return ducts from the house is heated by the furnace and distributed back into the house by the supply ducts. Most of the dust in a residential system is in the return side. *Tom Feiza, Mr. Fix-It, Inc.*

► Air Conveyance Systems

Do: General

_____ Have an HVAC (heating, ventilation, and air conditioning) technician do the following

    _____ Check to see that the blower cabinets, filter holders, and ducts are airtight.

    _____ Seal the ductwork as needed.

    _____ Be sure ducts aren't kinked or disconnected.

    _____ Make sure the blower cabinet has a bottom and any holes are sealed with aluminum tape.

_____ Determine the source of a leak if there is rust in the blower cabinet.

_____ Clean a soiled blower or blower cabinet.

_____ Replace any stained or soiled insulation in the blower cabinet.

_____ Be sure there is adequate flooring and lighting for access to mechanical equipment in an attic.

Ducts

Do

_____ To inspect the cleanliness of the ducts, remove a supply register or return grille and look in with a mirror and flashlight.

_____ Have your ducts professionally cleaned if they contain construction debris or more than 1/16 of an inch of dust.

_____ Otherwise, have your ducts cleaned once every five to ten years.

_____ Hire qualified professionals who belong to the National Air Duct Cleaners Association (NADCA) to clean your air conveyance system.

_____ Be sure to check their references.

_____ Only install ultraviolet (UV) lights in a system that is new or entirely free of dust.

_____ There must still be a pleated media filter (minimum of MERV-8) in the system. (See "Filtration" later in this section.)

OTHER VOICES: A CASE STUDY

One poor woman in Texas hired a company to clean her ducts for the advertised special of $99. When the crew arrived, they told her that her entire duct system was full of mold and recommended a $500 cleanup procedure. She paid them to do the work. In the weeks that followed, her duct system developed a musty smell. Her insurance agent inspected the system and told her that her ducts were not metal, but rather made of rigid fiberglass duct board.

Fiberglass duct board has aluminum foil on the outside, but the exposed internal surfaces are made of porous fiberglass and should never be cleaned with brushes. The entire duct system was ruined. It cost the homeowner over $3,500 to replace it—a bit more than the $99 special!

JEFF'S GEMS

It's important to check references, because there are always a few duct cleaners who take advantage of people's concerns. One of the ways some duct cleaners increase their profits is to offer you an antimicrobial or sanitizing treatment of the ducts near the end of the cleaning job, after they have earned your confidence. This treatment is unnecessary, so I recommend that you politely decline the offer.

Filtration

Do

_____ Check with manufacturers and/or installers on the compatibility of any filter for your HVAC system and how often the filter should be changed.

_____ Only use throw-away, pleated media filters with a MERV rating of at least an 8.

_____ Replace the filter at least once a year.

_____ Check that the filter holder is airtight.

_____ If you can see the cardboard edge of an installed filter, temporarily seal the access opening with duct tape.

_____ Measure the filter holder to be sure that the filter you are using is neither too large nor too small for the holder.

_____ Check that there are no sheet metal screws blocking easy installation and removal of the filter.

_____ Improve your filtration if the fan coil in the AC system has overflowed due to clogging of the condensate line.

Spending money to upgrade filtration in a heating or cooling system is one of the best investments you can make to improve IAQ. Good filtration cleans the air, but more importantly, it also helps to keep the equipment clean and reduces the chance of mold growth in the fan coil. The simplest upgrade is a one-inch pleated media filter with a MERV-8 rating. The next upgrade would be a thicker filter — two, four, or six inches thick — with a MERV rating of up to 11. These filters, however, require installation of a separate filter holder. The only HEPA filter available for a residential system is a bypass HEPA filter — an add-on with its own blower and case. I do not recommend such filters because they are expensive and only clean a small percentage of the return air.

Don't
_____ Install inexpensive fiberglass filters that you can see through.
_____ Use electronic or electrostatic filters, which have to be cleaned often.

Central Air Conditioning Only

Do
_____ Have an HVAC technician do the following:
  _____ Clean a soiled AC coil.
  _____ Check to see that water or slime is not accumulating in the condensate pan.
    _____ Clean the condensate pan and drain line as needed.
  _____ Replace any soiled fibrous insulation in the supply plenum (the enclosure from which the supply ducts exit).
  _____ Install an overflow tray with a float switch shut-off beneath an attic AC air handler.
_____ If an air handler unit used only for cooling is in the attic, close off the return grille(s) and supply registers during the heating season when the AC is not operating.

_____ Remember to open the return grilles and supply registers before operating the AC system.

_____ If you have a mini-split AC system with a washable plastic filter in the indoor unit, cut MERV-7 filter material to fit over the intake.

JEFF'S GEMS FOR HVAC TECHNICIANS

Do

_____ *Insulate at the exterior any ductwork that passes through an unconditioned space.*

_____ *Whenever possible in new construction, run ducts through conditioned space.*

_____ *Replace contaminated flexible ducts and rigid fiberglass duct board.*

_____ *Wherever possible, use all-metal duct systems with exterior insulation.*

_____ *Replace any flexible ducts if the outer gray wrap has disintegrated, allowing the interior fiberglass insulation to peel away from the clear, interior hose.*

_____ *Always clean the blower cabinet, blower, and air conditioning coil when cleaning ducts.*

_____ *Replace fiberglass insulation lining the air handler or ducts if the insulation is dirty and has gotten wet or moldy.*

_____ *Moisten moldy insulation before removal to prevent the aerosolization of dust into the surroundings as well as the system.*

_____ *Clean soiled diffusers.*

_____ *For liners, install nonfibrous insulation or fiberglass with aluminum-foil covering.*

_____ *In the air handler, use insulation that has a smooth surface and can easily be vacuumed or wiped clean.*

_____ *Abandon a duct system that is in a slab-on-grade and replace it with an overhead duct system.*

_____ *Handle dust from any components with caution (if clients have allergies or asthma).*

Don't

_____ *Have ductwork pass through concrete in contact with the ground.*

_____ *Place a return grille in the ceiling outside a bathroom. (Warm, moist air rising up from the bathroom can condense inside the cooler duct and fuel mold growth in the dust within.)*

_____ *Allow a condensate pan to overflow and water to leak out of an AC.*

_____ *Install exposed fibrous insulation in an air handler.*

_____ *Install duct board or other ducts with exposed fibrous insulation.*

_____ *Spray bactericide or fungicide into any part of an air conveyance system unless the product is EPA-approved for such use.*

_____ *Install a UV lamp to cure an IAQ problem in a dirty system.*

_____ *Use wall cavities or joist bays as returns (if clients have allergies or asthma).*

CONNIE'S COMMENTS

We included this advice so you could talk to HVAC technicians about these issues. And just in case you didn't know, a "conditioned" space means that it is heated and/or cooled.

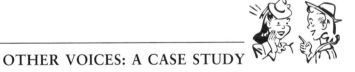

OTHER VOICES: A CASE STUDY

In slab homes and in both commercial and residential buildings, I have seen ducts in concrete that was poured on soil, or ducts partially in concrete and partially in the soil, or ducts buried in the soil or sand under the concrete. These types of installations are always a problem and should be avoided, because the ducts are in cool, damp environments and mold inevitably grows in the accumulated dust within the ducts. Sometimes the ducts even fill partially with water.

In one office I investigated, a periodic thumping noise came from the supply ducts when the heat or AC was running. The ducts were half filled with water, and the sound was caused by waves as they periodically blocked the air flow in the ducts. The ducts were so corroded that sand was pouring in — water and sand meeting, just like at the beach! The duct system was serving as a great humidifier. It was winter, and air exiting the ducts had a relative humidity (RH) of 75%. Water was condensing on all the windows in the building. Mold was growing on walls and in carpeting.

Portable Air Conditioners

Do

_____ If there is a slide-in, slide-out, washable plastic filter present, cut MERV-7 filter material to fit over the intake as additional filtration. (MERV stands for "minimum efficiency reporting value.")

➤ Other Kinds of Heating Systems

Electric Heat

Do

_____ Keep the indoor temperature 60°F or higher during the heating season, whether you are home or not.
_____ Keep the space around kick-space heaters accessible and clean.
_____ Periodically HEPA vacuum (use a vacuum cleaner with high efficiency particulate arrestance filtration) electric baseboard heaters.

Don't

_____ Turn electric heat in a basement or a room over a cold crawl space or garage down below 60°F.

Steam and Hot-Water Heat

Do

_____ Ask a technician to check that
_____ Steam radiators are pitched toward the valves.
_____ Steam radiator air vents open to allow air out but close as soon as the radiators fill with steam.

_____ Use a 36-inch crevice tool, attached to a HEPA vacuum, to clean radiators and baseboard convectors before the start of every heating season. (See www.midamericavacuum.com or www.vacuumstore.com.)

_____ Keep the enclosure around kick-space heaters in kitchens and bathrooms accessible and clean.

_____ Know where the water shut-off valves are for your boiler (as well as your water main).

_____ Label the valves.

Don't

_____ Paint steam radiator air vents.

➤ Humidification

Central Humidification

Do

_____ Use a trickle-type humidifier with a metal-mesh evaporative pad and *no* water reservoir, or use a steam humidifier (expensive but effective).

_____ Replace the metal evaporative pad annually.

_____ If the moisture source is in a duct, have a transparent glass or Lexan observation port installed in the duct.

_____ Check the glass or port periodically for stains or water in the bottom of the inside of the duct.

_____ If you see stains or water, call a technician to find out if repairs are needed.

_____ In a cold climate, keep the relative humidity under 40% in winter.

_____ Keep the RH even lower if you see condensation on your windows. (Monitor the RH with a thermo-hygrometer.)

_____ During the heating season, check all humidification equipment monthly for leaks.

_____ During the cooling season, always drain and shut down a central humidifier if you have central AC.

Don't

_____ In a cold climate, install a furnace humidifier in an attic.

_____ Use a rotating evaporative pad or spray central humidifier.

Portable Humidifiers

Do

_____ Check around any humidifier to make sure it's not leaking, particularly if there's carpeting.

_____ Operate a room humidifier that has a humidistat, which turns the humidifier on and off depending on the setting.

_____ Follow the manufacturer's directions for cleaning and maintaining a portable humidifier.

_____ In a cold climate, keep the relative humidity under 40% in winter and even lower if water is condensing on windows.

_____ Monitor the RH with a thermo-hygrometer.

Don't

_____ Use evaporative-pad or ultra-sonic portable humidifiers.

OTHER VOICES: Q & A

Q: What's the deal with humidifiers? Some say never use them because they grow mold and bacteria. Others who live in cold climates say that if the relative humidity falls below 30% in the winter, sinus membranes will dry out. What do you recommend?

A: Relative humidity under 30% in the colder months can be uncomfortable for many people. The danger, though, is that if you over-humidify, condensation will occur on cold surfaces and lead to mildew growth. That's why I recommend that, when possible, the relative humidity should be maintained under 40% in the winter, that any humidifier be equipped with a humidistat, and that the temperature and relative humidity be monitored with a thermo-hygrometer — available in many hardware stores. In very cold weather, monitor windows. If the indoor surface of the window is below the dew point of the indoor air and moisture condenses on the glass, you will have to lower the relative humidity. (If you cannot lower the RH, install storm windows or replacement windows with insulated glass.) To be safe, the best advice is to keep the indoor winter RH at the lowest comfortable level possible.

➤ Central Dehumidification

Do

_____ Use a filter with a rating of MERV-7. MERV-8 is preferable; MERV-11 is better! (MERV means minimum efficiency reporting value.)

Don't

_____ Operate the dehumidifier in the heating season.

JEFF'S GEMS

In a central dehumidification system, the temperature of the cool air should ideally be controlled by a thermostat and the relative humidity controlled, independent of temperature, by a separate dehumidistat. That way, when certain spaces are not in use they can be dehumidified but not cooled unnecessarily, leading to savings in energy.

➤ Hot-Water Heaters

Do

_____ Place a battery-operated floor water alarm near the hot-water heater.

_____ Or, if you have a central alarm system, install a floor-water alarm that is wired into the system.

_____ Install a hot-water tank with a ten-year rather than a five-year warranty.

_____ Know where the water shut-off valves are for your hot-water heater, as well as for your water main.

_____ Label the valves.

_____ If your hot-water heater leaks, refer to Part I, Dilemma 1D, "Floods and Leaks," and Part I, Dilemma 2, "Confirmation and Remediation."

CONNIE'S COMMENTS

Our hot-water tank gave up the ghost a few months after we moved into our house. (We hadn't gotten around to having the tank replaced, which turned out to be a foolish move.) I was on the second floor at the time. When I went to the basement, I had to wear rubber boots to wade over to the hot-water tank and shut off its water supply. What a mess!

► For People with Allergies, Asthma, or Environmental Sensitivities

Do

_____ Use a pleated media filter in your furnace, such as an Aprilaire, Air Bear, Honeywell, or Trane with a MERV rating of 11. (These filters require installation of a separate filter holder because they are four to six inches thick, and most holders can only hold a one-inch thick filter.)

_____ If your air conveyance system has one or two large returns, use a fiberglass furnace filter as a pre-filter in the return grille.

_____ If your air conveyance system has a return in every room, have Filtrex pre-filtered return grilles installed. (See www.fxallergy products.com/.)

_____ If you are installing a new duct system, install Filtrex grilles on the supplies as well as on the returns.

_____ Ask HVAC technicians to set up containment when cleaning your air conveyance system or replacing ducts, the furnace, or air conditioning equipment.

_____ If possible, wash and disinfect a window air conditioner each year before the cooling season. (The exterior case must be removed and all electrical components covered with plastic or aluminum foil to protect them from the water flow. Do this work outdoors.)

Don't

_____ Operate an AC if it smells moldy.

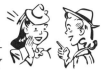

OTHER VOICES: A CASE STUDY

I heard about a family that hired a contractor to remove an old furnace — the kind that is sometimes called an "octopus" because it is big and has large ducts that radiate out from the furnace like the arms of an octopus. The old furnace and ducts were removed and a new furnace and ducts installed. Unfortunately, the people doing the work did not set up containment in the basement and were careless when handling the ducts and furnace, so moldy dust from the basement and from within the system spread into habitable spaces above. The homeowner and two of her children had mold sensitivities and experienced asthma symptoms, so the family had to move out of the house.

My Notes _____

_____

_____

_____

_____

_____

REMINDERS

1. UV lights or a HEPA bypass filter installed in a contaminated system will not solve the IAQ problems that can develop when microbial growth is disturbed by air flows.
2. If you aren't sure whether your air conveyance system is airtight, consult with an HVAC technician or a weatherization company.

WARNINGS

1. Filters you can see through are inadequate.
2. Rotating-pad evaporative humidifiers with a reservoir become contaminated with microbial growth.

3. *In a portable air conditioner, black dots on a background of gray house dust on the blower blades or walls of foam insulation behind the discharge grille are signs of mold growth.*

RELEVANT RESOURCES

Companies

Aprilaire manufactures a high-efficiency media filter. (800-334-6011, www.aprilaire.com).

Filtrex manufactures supply and return grilles with easily accessed filters that supplement the HVAC system's primary filter. (See fxallergyproducts.com/.)

Honeywell manufactures media filters (www.yourhome.honeywell.com).

An Institute that Trains and Certifies HVAC Professionals

National Air Duct Cleaners Association (NADCA), Washington, DC (202-737-2926, www.nadca.com).

An Organization

The American Society of Home Inspectors, Des Plaines, IL (800-743-2744, www.ashi.org).

Products

36-inch vacuum crevice tool: Available online; search for "crevice tool" and "vacuum cleaner," or see www.midamericavacuum.com or www.vacuumstore.com.

Dehumidifiers: Therma-Store in Madison, WI (800-533-7533, www.thermastor.com).

Hygrometer: Monitors relative humidity; available in many building supply stores and online. Therma-Stor sells a recording thermo-hygrometer (a hygrometer that also measures temperature) with an alarm (www.thermastor.com).

Media filters: Available in some building-supply stores and online. (See www.aprilaire.com, www.filtersamerica.com, www.filtersusa.com, www.oxyclean.com, or www.yourhome.honeywell.com.)

Publications

Building Air Quality: A Guide for Building Owners and Facility Managers, U.S. Environmental Protection Agency and the National Institute for Occupational Safety and Health, 1991.

"Should You Have the Air Ducts in Your Home Cleaned?" EPA 402-K-97-02, February 1991 (www.epa.gov/iaq/pubs/humidif.html or IAQ INFO, PO Box 37133, Washington, DC 20013-7133, 800-438-4318).

"Use and Care of Home Humidifiers—Indoor Air Facts No. 8," EPA 402-F-91-101, February 1991 (www.epa.gov/iaq/pubs/humidif.html or IAQ INFO, PO Box 37133, Washington, DC 20013-7133, 800-438-4318).

G. PROPERTY I WANT TO BUY OR RENT

_____ There's a musty smell in a property I want to buy or rent.
_____ There's visible mold in the property.
Where? _____
_____ A property I'm thinking of buying or renting has had mold removed.
_____ I was given a mold test report that I don't understand.
_____ I have other concerns. _____
_____
_____

Do
_____ Try to determine the source of a musty odor before moving in.
_____ Be suspicious if you see the following in a building you are considering living in:
        _____ Scented candles in certain rooms, particularly in below-grade spaces.
        _____ Plug-in fragrance emitters.
        _____ Abundant, fragrant flowers or potpourri indoors.
        _____ Scent sprays in rooms other than bathrooms.
_____ Ask that all fragrance emitters be removed from the property and the windows and doors closed for a day or so before you return for a "second sniff."

JEFF'S GEMS

Floral fragrances can mask the musty odors created by mold growth. It's possible that visible mold or a musty smell can be easy to remediate, but it's *also possible that there may be a major concealed mold problem requiring extensive and costly remediation.*

_____ Hire the best independent home inspector you can find and be sure he or she looks for any visible signs of moisture or leakage in a property you are thinking of renting or buying.

     _____ The American Society of Home Inspectors (www.ashi.org) has a geographic list of members.

_____ Follow the tips in Part I, Dilemma 1C, "The Rooms In Between" (especially in "Rooms with Water") for advice on how to find mold growth.

JEFF'S GEMS

Some people want air testing for mold spores to be a routine part of real estate transactions. Mold grows indoors because of moisture problems caused by leaks, high humidity, and water intrusion due to foundation or grading problems. These are all issues that should be identified through a thorough, visual building inspection and assessment, not through air testing. Air test conditions can be conducive to inaccurate results, particularly in the tense and often crowded atmosphere of a real estate transaction. (See Part I, Dilemma 2A, "Testing for Mold.") Furniture owned by the occupant may contain mold growth, a termite inspector may be walking around inside with clothing covered with mold spores from a crawl space, and occupants may be opening doors that should remain closed—such as a door leading from the first floor to a moldy basement. And even if test results that declare a space "mold free" are accurate, mold can grow within 24 to 48 hours if the conditions are right. So a space can be mold-free one week and a mold farm the next. A reassuring, valid mold test is only a statement of conditions in that space at that time. Not much help to someone who is moving in weeks or even months later!

However, mold testing can be useful in investigating a suspected mold problem. If a property smells musty or you think mold growth may be pres-

ent, it makes sense to have an IAQ professional undertake air and dust sampling prior to occupancy, but be sure that the report will attempt to pinpoint the source of a problem.

_____ Hire an IAQ professional to help you figure out why mold is growing, how extensive the mold growth is, and what should be done to get rid of it.

_____ Require that the mold problem be eradicated before moving in.

    _____ Obtain a copy of the remediation proposal.

    _____ Request photographs of the remediated areas, showing the extent of contamination and progress of the cleanup.

    _____ Obtain copies of any pre- and post-remediation mold testing.

    _____ For a second opinion, consider having someone *you* hire do post-remediation testing. (See Part I, Dilemma 2, "Confirmation and Remediation.")

_____ Solve any mold problem present before putting a property you own up for sale or rent.

► For People with Allergies, Asthma, or Environmental Sensitivities

Do

_____ Have an IAQ professional check below-grade spaces for mold growth before committing to a property.

_____ Unless you must have cooling for health reasons, avoid purchasing or renting a property that has forced hot-air heat or central air conditioning if the house has been previously occupied, because the HVAC (heating, ventilation, and air conditioning) system may be contaminated with allergens.

_____ Spend at least an hour or two at the property to see if you experience symptoms.

_____ Eliminate all carpeting in below-grade spaces and replace with ceramic tile or vinyl. (See Part I, Dilemma 1A, "My Basement.")

_____ If you can afford it, replace all the carpets in the home with solid flooring.

Don't

_____ Purchase or rent a property that has a musty odor.

_____ Rent property with old wall-to-wall carpeting or with carpeting that smells musty.

My Notes _____

_____

_____

_____

_____

_____

OTHER VOICES: Q & A

Q: We are buying a house that is under construction. The house is being framed but it hasn't been closed in yet. A recent deluge of snow and rain makes me worry about mold. Do you think the framing may have gotten moldy? If so, what can we do about it?

A: I wouldn't worry too much, because mold growth would be minimal in cold weather. Still, the framing should be kept open so it can dry out. Don't forget to check the basement, which can get wet during construction when it rains or snows. If there are puddles of water in the basement, have them mopped up and the basement aired out. In a home being built during warm, humid weather, a basement that has gotten damp may have to be isolated from the exterior and habitable rooms above (by closing doors and windows) and be dehumidified. If you are still concerned, have several joists or studs, especially in the basement, surface tested for mold.

REMINDER

In some states, disclosure of prior or current mold problems is required in real estate transactions.

WARNING

If you are considering moving into a property and there are many scented candles or fragrance emitters present, the owner may be concealing the musty smell of a mold problem.

CONNIE'S COMMENTS

This is a short section but an important one. You don't want to move into a property and then find out it has a serious mold problem!

RELEVANT RESOURCES

Institutes That Train and/or Certify Mold and Indoor Air Quality Professionals

American Conference of Governmental Industrial Hygienists (ACGIH), Cincinnati, OH (513-742-2020, www.acgih.org).

American Indoor Air Quality Council (AIAQC), Glendale, AZ (800-942-0832, www.iaqcouncil.org).

American Industrial Hygiene Association (AIHA), Fairfax, VA (703-849-8888, www.aiha.org).

Association of Energy Engineers (AEE), Atlanta, GA (770-447-5083, www.aeecenter.org).

Indoor Air Quality Association (IAQA), Rockville, MD (301-231-8388, www.iaqa.org).

An Organization

American Society of Home Inspectors, Des Plaines, IL (800-743-2744, www.ashi.org).

H. HOTELS AND AUTOMOBILES

_____ A hotel room smells moldy.
_____ My car smells musty.

_____ I have other concerns. _____
_____
_____
_____

JEFF'S GEMS

Hotel rooms and cars can have IAQ problems just the way other inside spaces can. You don't have much control over conditions in a hotel or car, but there are still some steps you can take to protect your health when you travel.

Do

_____ Place a water-impervious mat that can be cleaned or replaced over carpeting in front of the driver and passenger seats.

_____ After driving in the rain, using a mirror and flashlight check the underside of the dashboard for dripping water.

_____ Use the *paper-towel test* on automobile carpeting to see if the carpet is the source of a musty odor.

JEFF'S GEMS

The paper-towel test *is a handy and relatively easy way to figure out if a surface is emitting a smell. Place a piece of odorless paper towel, folded in half twice, over the area in question. Then cover the paper towel with a flat piece of aluminum foil. Use removable painter's tape to secure the edges of the foil to the surface. Leave the foil-covered paper towel in place for 24 to 48 hours. Remove the "assembly," folding the towel into the foil so that it is completely covered and sealed on both sides. Take the wrapped paper towel outside and, without uncovering it, loosen an edge of the foil and cautiously take a sniff. If the surface on which the towel rested is emitting an odor, the towel should have adsorbed (taken up) some of the chemicals causing the smell.*

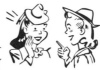

OTHER VOICES: A CASE STUDY

One woman called me from Virginia with an odd story about a musty-smelling car. Her car had been rear-ended at a red light and had been repaired at a collision shop. She inspected the car and found that the carpeting under the backseat was damp and the trunk contained several inches of water. I never saw the car, but it seems likely that the damage was not properly repaired, and rainwater was dripping into the trunk around the edges, leading to mold growth in the carpet dust. I recommended that the family make the trunk leak-tight, replace all the carpeting in the car, clean the upholstery, and have the heating and air conditioning professionally disinfected.

➤ For People with Allergies, Asthma, or Environmental Sensitivities

Do

_____ Stay in a hotel with windows that can open.

_____ If a hotel room smells musty, try another room or find another hotel.

_____ Place extra sheets or carpet protector (www.pro-tect.com), an adhesive-backed plastic, on a hotel room carpet to create "paths," so foot traffic will not aerosolize (make airborne) irritants and allergens.

_____ Run an automobile's heating or cooling system with the blower on high for 20 seconds with the windows open, to air out the system before you set off on your trip.

_____ Use the heat and AC on recirculate to prevent outdoor airborne debris from being deposited on the car's cooling coil.

_____ When you purchase a new car, get one that has a cabin air filter, if possible.

_____ Carry a NIOSH N95 mask with you when you travel.

Don't

_____ Stay in a carpeted ground-floor room in a motel.

_____ Operate a musty-smelling hotel or motel room air conditioner or heating unit.

_____ Let the housekeeping staff clean the hotel room while you are staying there, because they may disturb moldy dust.

_____ Let anyone introduce fragrances into an automobile's heating/air conditioning system as part of cleaning and maintenance.

CONNIE'S COMMENTS

When we travel by car, Jeff and I take a roll of Pro-Tect carpet protector with us. It's a little cumbersome to drag the roll around, but it's worth it, because once we cover the walked-on areas of the carpet in a hotel room, he stops coughing.

My Notes _____

_____

_____

_____

_____

_____

_____

REMINDERS

1. *Whenever possible, stay in a hotel with operable windows.*
2. *Don't settle for a musty-smelling hotel room.*

WARNING

Housekeeping staff in a hotel can disturb moldy carpet dust or use an unfiltered vacuum cleaner that spews out allergens in its exhaust.

Products

Carpet covering (self-adhering clear plastic): Pro-tect Associates, Inc., Northfield, IL
(800-545-0826, www.pro-tect.com).

NIOSH N95 double-strap, fine-particle mask: Available in most hardware and
building supply stores. Brands include 3M #8210 and Gerson #1710.

A Publication

Your Car Can Be Hazardous to Your Health, Basil M. Rudusky. Bloomington, IN:
AuthorHouse, 2002.

I. OUTSIDE THE BUILDING

_____ There is green stuff on my driveway or sidewalk that I think is mold.

_____ I have moldy leaves in my yard.

_____ My deck gets slippery in the rain.

_____ There is black mildew on the siding.

_____ There are mushrooms growing on the outside of the building.

_____ I have other concerns. _____

_____

_____

OTHER VOICES: A CASE STUDY

At a three-year-old condominium complex at a coastal location in the Carolinas, unit owners were astonished to find large mushrooms growing out of the siding above the door trim beneath a large upper-level deck. On the three-level decks in each of several buildings in the complex, a metal flashing had been left out at a small gap between horizontal boards that caught rainwater. Since the day of construction, all the rainwater that collected on top of these boards had flowed into the small gap and leaked down behind the siding. The vertical posts near the decks that supported the building corners, built of two-by-six lumber and concealed by the siding, were so rotted that the wood could be scooped out by hand.

If you see mushrooms sprouting on your siding, call in a professional home inspector (www.ashi.org) who uses moisture meters to give you guidance on the extent of the problem and what you can do about it.

Algae and moss, both green in color, are signs of excess moisture — too much water collecting on walkways and driveways or too much rainwater running down the exterior walls or splashing onto them. Dampness in wood can lead to mold problems and rot, but algae and moss are not mold and do not themselves rot wood.

Do

_____ Trim bushes and other ground-level plants at least eighteen inches away from the exterior of the building.

_____ To prevent splash that will decay siding and sliding doors, add a gutter to any roof that drains onto a deck, stoop, or landing.

_____ Check the outside of the building during a heavy rain to make sure roof run-off isn't flowing down the exterior surfaces.

_____ Keep exterior water off the siding by having a clean, well-maintained gutter system or an adequate overhang (at least 18 inches).

_____ Make sure that all the drip-cap flashings, also called "Z" flashings, on top of exterior windows and doors, as well as any decorative, horizontal trim on the siding, are sloped away from and not toward the building.

_____ Hire a home inspector or building consultant who will look for stains and use a moisture meter to detect dampness under windows or in ceilings under the roof.

      _____ If dampness or stains are found, have the inspector help you figure out where rainwater is getting into the building. (See Part I, Dilemma 1C, "The Rooms In Between.")

Don't

_____ Allow any lawn-sprinkler water to spray the exterior of the house.

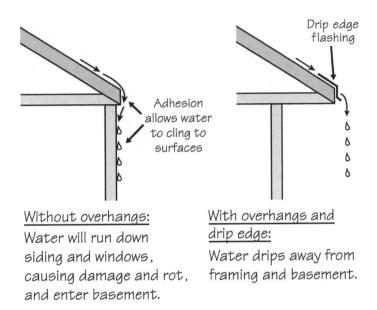

Drip edge flashing

Adhesion allows water to cling to surfaces

<u>Without overhangs:</u>
Water will run down siding and windows, causing damage and rot, and enter basement.

<u>With overhangs and drip edge:</u>
Water drips away from framing and basement.

In cities most homes have gutters, but in rural areas gutters are less common. A good roof overhang protects the siding, windows, and doors from water flows where gutters are not installed. *Tom Feiza, Mr. Fix-It, Inc.*

_____ Let ivy or branches from plantings come in contact with wood siding or trim.

_____ Allow branches to touch the roof.

_____ Allow tree branches to extend over a roof or gutter system.

_____ Allow roof water to splash onto a deck.

My Notes _____

_____

_____

_____

_____

REMINDER

Rainwater from roofs, gutters, or downspouts should never stream down the exterior of a building.

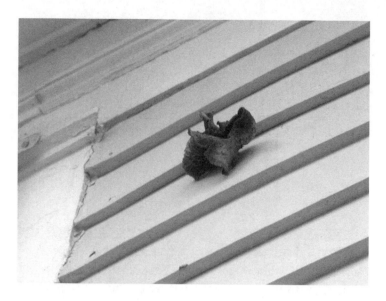

The mushroom appeared on the pressed-wood siding at the outside of a bedroom. There were no stains at the inside of the house, but water was leaking through a small hole at the edge of the roofing into the exterior part of the wall. The siding was constantly wet, and wood behind the siding was being rotted by hidden macrofungal growth which became visible when the mushroom sprouted. *May Indoor Air Investigations LLC*

 WARNING

Mushroom growth can signal hidden water and mold problems that can cause paint to peel on the exterior and siding and sheathing to rot.

RELEVANT RESOURCES

An Organization

The American Society of Home Inspectors, Des Plaines, IL (800-743-2744, www.ashi.org).

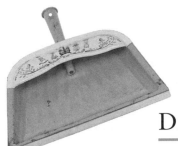

DILEMMA 2

Confirmation and Remediation

JEFF'S GEMS

Air testing for mold spores can easily overlook or underestimate a mold problem, particularly if at the time the air is sampled, no one happens to be walking on a moldy carpet or moving moldy books. Air testing for mold spores is an important tool, but only when the results are accurate and lead the way to the sources *of mold contamination.*

Sometimes a building occupant can get rid of a mold problem, if the problem is small and no one in the building is sensitized to mold. Sometimes, however, a mold problem must be remediated by professionals.

RELEVANT RESOURCES

A Publication

Guidelines on Assessment and Remediation of Fungi in Indoor Environments. New York: New York City Department of Health and Mental Hygiene, Bureau of Environmental and Occupational Disease Epidemiology, 2000 (www.lchd .org/environhealth/aq/pdfs/NYC%20DOH%20Guidelines.pdf).

A. TESTING FOR MOLD

_____ I'm wondering if mold testing should be done.

_____ If so, should I test for mold myself?

_____ Or should I hire a professional?

_____ Mold testing has been done, and I don't know what the report means.

_____ Mold test results declare that the air quality is fine, and yet I'm still experiencing symptoms indoors.

_____ I have other concerns. _____

_____

_____

JEFF'S GEMS

When professionals test for mold, they may gather air as well as dust samples that are then analyzed by a lab. The results may be reported quantitatively, as the concentration of a particular type of spore per cubic meter of air, or qualitatively, as low, medium, or high concentrations. Quantitative results are usually required in legal cases. Total spore testing counts all spores, dead and alive. Culturable spore testing only counts spores that are alive. Home test kits only test for live spores.

Reassuring results from culturable spore testing or home test kits may not mean much to people with mold sensitivities, because in many indoor environments, most spores are dead but still allergenic.

► Testing on My Own

Do

_____ Find the source of the mold if you use a home mold test kit (available in many hardware and building supply stores) and the results are positive. (See Part I, Dilemma 1, "Mold, Inside and Out.")

_____ If you cannot find the mold growth, hire an IAQ professional to help you.

Don't

_____ Assume that negative test results from a home mold test kit mean there is no mold problem present.

➤ Hiring Professionals to Test

Do

_____ When considering hiring professionals to sample for mold

     _____ Ask for references.

     _____ Ask to see a sample of a report.

         _____ If you don't understand the report, ask the tester or another IAQ professional to explain the results to you.

     _____ Require proof of training or certification.

_____ Ask for a copy of the professional mold test report if mold testing has already been conducted in the building.

     _____ If you don't understand the report, confer with an IAQ professional.

Don't

_____ Trust test results that say there is no problem when people are having symptoms in an indoor environment.

➤ For People with Allergies, Asthma, or Environmental Sensitivities

Do

_____ Show a mold test report to your physician if you are experiencing symptoms or have mold allergies or sensitivities.

My Notes _____

_____

_____

_____

_____

_____

OTHER VOICES: Q & A

Q: I bought a settle-plate home mold test kit. The lab results came back saying there was mold in every room. What should I do next?

A: A settle plate is a plastic dish containing nutrients for mold growth. Many IAQ professionals think that the settle-plate test you used is a poor indicator of indoor mold problems, because there are always mold spores in indoor air. (Many of these spores may enter the building from outdoors.) Mold colonies will therefore almost always grow on the settle plate. Have the testing redone by a professional and the results analyzed by a qualified lab. If the second test confirms your original results, hire an IAQ investigator to find the sources of airborne contaminants, and if indoors, a remediator to eradicate them.

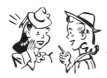

OTHER VOICES: CASE STUDIES

One man hired a "professional" mold investigator who did not have much training or practical experience and who took one air sample in the bathroom and another outdoors for comparison. The concentration of one type of mold spore in the bathroom was 50% higher than the concentration of that type of mold outdoors. Based on this data, the professional recommended that the tiled bathroom be demolished — at a $15,000 cost — and said a friend of his could do the work.

The homeowner called me for a second opinion and sent me the original test results, which told me that the spores found in the sample were only produced by mushrooms. I asked the homeowner whether there were any mushrooms growing out of the tile. No, he replied. The spores, common in outdoor air, had probably come into the room through an open window and settled into the dust in the bath mat. I suggested that he wash the bath mat: a much cheaper solution to the problem!

Another family was ready to burn their house down because an incompetent mold tester took samples in a home after disturbing moldy dust in a basement while the door leading to the first floor was open. The entire house was briefly contaminated with basement spores, so when the tester took an air sample upstairs, it appeared as though the entire house was moldy. Several days later, I took an air sample upstairs before opening the door leading to the basement, and the concentration of spores was only slightly elevated. The basement needed to be professionally remediated, but the rest of the house only needed a thorough HEPA vacuuming (using a vacuum cleaner with high efficiency particulate arrestance filtration).

A similar situation occurred during a real estate transaction. A tester took an air sample in a child's bedroom after he disturbed dust in a very moldy attic and left open the pull-down stairway in the hall adjacent to the child's room. The mold spore levels in the child's room were so high that the homeowner feared for the health of his child. A few days later, I sampled the home before opening the attic hatch and found virtually no attic spores in the bedroom air. The attic had a mold problem and had to be professionally remediated, but the buyers were so spooked by what they perceived as a house that was completely contaminated that they withdrew their offer. The sellers ended up replacing the entire roof and all the attic insulation before they found another buyer for the home.

REMINDER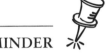

If you don't understand a mold-test report, confer with an IAQ professional.

WARNING

Do not make drastic decisions — such as spending thousands of dollars on remediation or vacating a property — based on the results of a settle-plate mold test.

RELEVANT RESOURCES

Institutes That Train and/or Certify Mold and Indoor Air Quality Professionals

American Conference of Governmental Industrial Hygienists (ACGIH), Cincinnati, OH (513-742-2020, www.acgih.org).

American Indoor Air Quality Council (AIAQC), Glendale, AZ (800-942-0832, www.iaqcouncil.org).

American Industrial Hygiene Association (AIHA), Fairfax, VA (703-849-8888, www.aiha.org).

Association of Energy Engineers (AEE), Atlanta, GA (770-447-5083, www.aeecenter.org).

Indoor Air Quality Association (IAQA), Rockville, MD (301-231-8388, www.iaqa.org).

Laboratories That Sell Test Kits and Analyze Dust Samples from Carpets and Other Surfaces

Aerotech Labs, Phoenix, AZ (800-651-4802, www.aerotechpk.com).

DACI Laboratory, Johns Hopkins University Asthma and Allergy Center, Baltimore, MD (800-344-3224, www.hopkinsmedicine.org/allergy/daci/index.html).

Envirologix, Portland, ME (866-408-4597, http://envirologix.com), also sells test kits for mycotoxins.

Northeast Laboratory, Winslow, ME (800-244-8378, www.nelabservices.com).

B. CLEANING IT UP MYSELF

———— I don't know whether I should clean up mold myself or hire a professional to do the work.

———— If I decide to tackle the job, how do I go about accomplishing the task?

———— Once the mold is removed, will it grow back?

———— I have other concerns. ——————————————————

————————————————————————————————————

————————————————————————————————————

————————————————————————————————————

————————————————————————————

JEFF'S GEMS

Small mold cleanup jobs, defined by the New York City Department of Health and Mental Hygiene, Bureau of Environmental and Occupational Disease

Epidemiology as "ten square feet or less" of mold growth,[*] *can be tackled by occupants as long as no one in the house or work space is allergic or sensitized to mold. Larger mold problems, as well as mold growing in areas flooded with "black water" (water tainted with human waste), must be cleaned up by professionals.*

Refer to Part I, Dilemma 1D, "Floods and Leaks," for cleaning advice specific to leaks and floods, and Part I, Dilemma 1F, "Heating and Cooling Systems," for cleaning and maintenance advice specific to mechanical systems.

➤ Bathrooms

Do

_____ Wearing protective gloves and eye protection, get rid of musty odors from a sink by carefully pouring a weak solution of water and bleach (approximately one part bleach to ten parts water) into the sink overflow hole.

_____ Wash or replace shower curtains that have visible mold growth.

➤ The Kitchen

Do

_____ Wearing protective gloves and eye protection, pour a dilute solution of water and bleach (approximately one part bleach to ten parts water) down the disposer to remove smells.

    _____ Rinse thoroughly before turning the disposer on.

    _____ Stand back from the sink when you first turn the disposer on.

_____ Wearing protective gloves and eye protection, clean moldy gaskets in the refrigerator door with diluted bleach (approximately one part bleach to ten parts water).

_____ Replace gaskets that are moldy and split.

---

[*] *Guidelines on Assessment and Remediation of Fungi in Indoor Environments* (New York: New York City Department of Health and Mental Hygiene, Bureau of Environmental and Occupational Disease Epidemiology, 2000), 8–10.

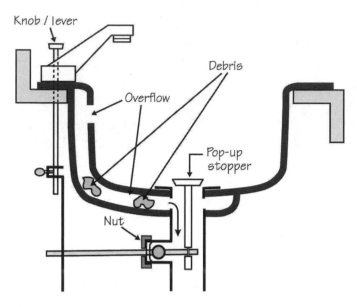

Knob / lever

Debris

Overflow

Pop-up stopper

Nut

Overflow hole is connected to drain line below sink. Debris can collect out of sight in overflow chamber and cause a smell.

Depending on just how moist and dirty conditions are in the overflow, bacteria and/or mold can grow. The odor can vary from a sour-sponge smell to a musty smell. *Tom Feiza, Mr. Fix-It, Inc.*

► Personal Possessions and Furnishings

_____ Air out musty-smelling or moldy sheets and blankets in the sun.

_____ Then wash or dry-clean the sheets and blankets as appropriate.

_____ Wash or dry-clean musty-smelling clothing.

_____ Wash or dry-clean musty-smelling window treatments.

_____ Clean moldy leather goods (preferably outdoors) with leather soap, and then polish the items.

_____ Throw out moldy or musty-smelling cardboard boxes.

_____ HEPA vacuum (use a vacuum with high efficiency particulate arrestance filtration) outdoors any books that smell musty but do not contain visible mold.

_____ Confer with a book dealer for advice on how to clean a moldy but valuable book.

► Regular Household Cleaning

_____ Use a HEPA vacuum or a central vacuum cleaning system (but only if it exhausts to the exterior) rather than a regular vacuum cleaner or wet/dry vac.
_____ Use dehumidification to help dry carpets after they've been cleaned.
_____ Replace musty-smelling sponges and mops.

Solid Surfaces

_____ Clean smaller patches of mold on walls or ceilings with a regular household cleaner suited for the purpose.
    _____ Test a small spot on the surface first to be sure the cleaning agent doesn't cause damage.
    _____ Run a fan in the window on exhaust while cleaning, or isolate the area by closing doors that lead to other rooms.
    _____ While cleaning, wear protective gear, including a properly fitted mask with a minimum NIOSH (National Institute of Occupational Safety and Health) rating of N95 and long protective gloves.
    _____ HEPA vacuum surfaces in the room when you are finished removing the mold.
_____ Have moldy ceiling tiles replaced.
    _____ To better control moldy dust, lightly spray the tiles with water containing a small amount of detergent before removing them.
_____ To clean an unfinished surface of wood furniture that contains mold
    _____ Wipe the surface with a rag moistened with denatured or isopropyl (rubbing) alcohol.
    _____ Wear gloves and eye protection.
    _____ Refer to manufacturer's precautions for use of the alcohol.
    _____ Seal the surface with a thin coat of clear shellac or varnish.
        _____ If the varnish is oil-based, wait for the alcohol to dry completely.
_____ Clean the finished surfaces of wood furniture with a suitable cleaning agent and then wax or polish.
_____ Clean wood furniture outside if possible.

_____ If you must do this work inside

        _____ Cover other surfaces to protect them from moldy dust.

        _____ Ventilate well by operating a fan on exhaust.

        _____ Have a fire extinguisher handy. (The alcohol is combustible.)

        _____ HEPA vacuum the room when the work is completed.

Don't

_____ Use undiluted bleach for cleaning.

_____ Use a bleach solution if the smell of bleach bothers you or someone else who lives in your home, or if bleach irritates your skin.

_____ Have carpets washed during humid weather.

_____ Keep leather goods that contain extensive mildew growth.

_____ Keep thick clothing that still smells musty after being washed or dry-cleaned.

_____ Keep upholstered furniture, mattresses, or pillows that contain visible mold or smell musty.

_____ Clean surfaces with sour- or musty-smelling sponges or mops.

CONNIE'S COMMENTS

If you used a sour-smelling sponge and now the surface you wiped has acquired that smell, rinse the surface with a mild ammonia and water solution or with a baking soda and water mixture.

_____ Cover up a musty smell with a fragranced spray, candle, or plug-in fragrance emitter.

_____ Depend on an air purifier to get rid of a musty smell.

_____ Use alcohol near an open flame (gas stove, wood stove, or fireplace).

_____ Depressurize (use a fan on exhaust) in a room that contains combustion equipment. (This can cause backdrafting of combustion products, including carbon monoxide.)

► For People with Allergies, Asthma, or Environmental Sensitivities

Do

_____ Consult with your physician before tackling a mold problem.

_____ Preferably have someone else clean up the mold.

      _____ Be sure that person sets up containment. (See Part I, Dilemma 1A, "My Basement.")

           _____ Use ZipWall posts to erect fire retardant sheet-plastic walls around the area (www.zipwall.com).

           _____ Close all doors leading to other rooms and cover the closed doors with plastic sheeting.

      _____ Stay away from the space while this work is going on.

Don't

_____ Clean up mold yourself.

_____ Touch mold or work with hazardous cleaning liquids with bare hands.

_____ Apply shellac or varnish to furniture surfaces if you are chemically sensitive.

CONNIE'S COMMENTS

Don't panic about a small amount of mold on a ceiling, wall, or window. You can clean up small areas of mold like this if you're careful and if neither you nor anyone else in your home is sensitive to the stuff.

My Notes _____

_____

_____

_____

_____

_____

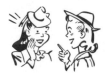

OTHER VOICES: Q & A

Q: The window air conditioner in our family room was leaking. A corner of the carpet soaked up the water and was wet for a long time before we realized it. We've fixed the air conditioner and had the carpet cleaned, but that area of the room still smells musty. I've read about various air purifiers and am wondering if this will help get rid of the smell.

A: Despite the fact that the carpet was cleaned, the lingering musty smell in that corner suggests that the carpet still contains moldy dust or bacteria and yeast colonies. There might also be mold-eating mites present, as well as silverfish hunting the mites and spiders hunting the silverfish—all leaving allergenic poop and body parts behind. Do you want your children crawling or walking on this jungle? I recommend that you remove the carpet and pad, HEPA vacuum and paint-seal the floor beneath, and either install new carpeting or, if anyone in your family has allergies, asthma, or any environmental sensitivities, install a tile or vinyl floor with an area rug on top if you want a softer surface.

As for the air purifier, such devices aren't effective as long as the source of contamination remains present—in this case, your moldy carpet.

REMINDER

After wall-to-wall carpets have been washed, dehumidify or ventilate the room with dry air by opening up windows and doors. (Don't do this on a rainy day or a hot, humid day.)

WARNING

Regular vacuum cleaners and wet/dry vacs can emit allergens in their exhaust.

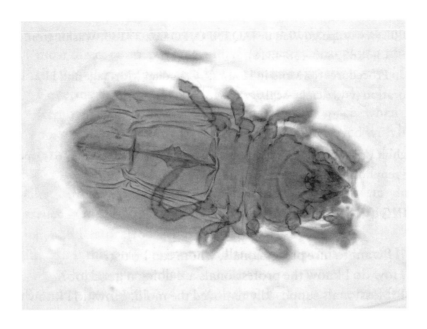

This skin was shed by a mold-eating, microscopic mite. You can see that there are a few leg pieces missing. I found this mite skin in a dust sample I took from a moldy baseboard in the finished basement of a beautiful Cape Cod vacation home, whose occupants suffered asthma symptoms. *May Indoor Air Investigations LLC*

Relevant Resources

Products

HEPA vacuum: Available at many home supply stores and online. (See
www.miele.com.)
NIOSH N95 mask: Available in many hardware and building supply stores. Brands
include 3M #8210 and Gerson #1710.
ZipWall: Adjustable posts used to set up a containment (www.zipwall.com,
800-718-2255).

Publications

"Biological Pollutants in Your Home," Consumer Public Safety Commission, Docu-
ment #425 (www.epa.gov/iaq or IAQ INFO, PO Box 37133, Washington,
DC 20013-7133, 800-438-4318).
"A Brief Guide to Mold, Moisture and Your Home," EPA 402-K-02-003, Summer

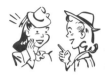

OTHER VOICES: A CASE STUDY

An allergist referred a female patient to me who had been plagued for several years by a chronic cough. She kept the habitable spaces in her home impeccably clean, and her finished, moldy basement had supposedly been remediated, but she still experienced symptoms that medication did not alleviate.

I took dust samples from clothing in her closets, as well as from rugs and pieces of cushioned furniture. The woman operated a very lucrative business from her home and spent many hours on the phone while she sat on an easy chair in the family room. The chair was contaminated with Aspergillus *mold (perhaps fueled by body moisture), and there were spores on her clothing in the closet—possibly from that chair. There was also some* Aspergillus *mold growth on furniture and doors in the basement that the remediators had missed.*

She eliminated the easy chair and some wool rugs, and had the moldy basement surfaces remediated. She also eliminated a feather quilt from her bed. (See Part II, Dilemma 3B, "Other Rooms and Their Contents.") Several weeks after she made these changes, her physician reported that the woman's health had improved significantly.

REMINDER

Hire the best remediator you can find and insist on containment.

WARNING

If you are still experiencing symptoms, even though the mold has supposedly been removed, your home may need further testing and remediation.

Institutes that Train and/or Certify Mold, Air Quality or Cleaning Professionals

American Conference of Governmental Industrial Hygienists (ACGIH), Cincinnati, OH (513-742-2020, www.acgih.org).

American Indoor Air Quality Council (AIAQC), Glendale, AZ (800-942-0832, www.iaqcouncil.org).

American Industrial Hygiene Association (AIHA), Fairfax, VA (703-849-8888, www.aiha.org).

Association of Energy Engineers (AEE), Atlanta, GA (770-447-5083, www.aeecenter.org).

Indoor Air Quality Association (IAQA), Rockville, MD (301-231-8388, www.iaqa.org).

Institute of Inspection, Cleaning, and Restoration Certification (IICRC), Vancouver, WA (800-835-4624, www.certifiedcleaners.org). Offers reference guide S520.

Restoration Consultants, Sacramento, CA (888-617-3266, www.restcon.com).

Restoration Industry Association (RIA), Columbia, MD (800-272-7012, www.ascr.org).

Organizations

American Conference of Governmental Industrial Hygienists, Cincinnati, OH (513-742-2020, www.acgih.org).

Carpet and Rug Institute, Dalton, GA (706-278-3176, www.carpet-rug.org).

A Product

Respirator mask: Available in some building supply stores as well as online. (See www.allergybegone.com.)

A Website

www.cdc.gov/niosh/docs/2003-144/ for information on different respirators and masks.

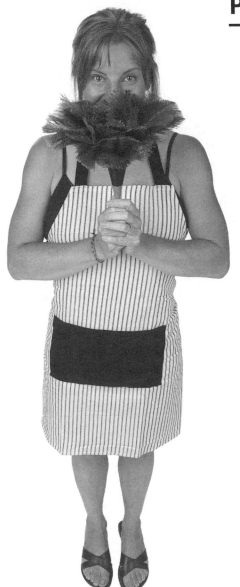

PART II

Problems Other Than Mold

This section of the book discusses a number of indoor contaminants, irritants, and allergens other than mold, including volatile organic compounds (VOCs), bacteria, pet dander, and dust mite allergens. The list of possibilities is long, as we mentioned in the Introduction. (There is some overlap between Parts I and II, because conditions conducive to mold growth can also be conducive to the growth of bacteria and yeast.) We are also including some tips about conditions not directly related to indoor air quality that can affect our physical comfort, such as heat.

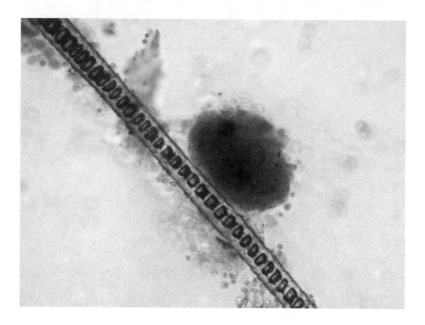

When you move into a new home, you can never be sure what is lurking in the carpets. In one home, a couple moved in with a child who was allergic to cats. I took a sample of the dust in the carpet covering the stairs leading to the basement and found cat dander and an insect fecal pellet. *May Indoor Air Investigations LLC*

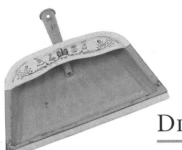

DILEMMA 3

What and Where?

In most modern, "tight" buildings, such as large residential complexes and hotels, offices, schools, courthouses, and hospitals, windows don't open, so we depend on the building's ventilation system to supply fresh air. All too often that system is poorly maintained, or the amount of fresh air being introduced into the building has been minimized to save on energy costs. The amount of fresh air can thus be insufficient to dilute and flush out contaminants, and many building occupants who are sensitized continue to suffer symptoms.

Although the windows in most homes are operable, they are rarely opened in many areas of the country, so the only fresh air introduced into the building enters through construction cracks around doors and windows. And the tighter the construction, the fewer the openings. This is not that different from a modern building with inoperable windows!

A. ROOMS WITH WATER

_____ A bathroom smells even when not in use.
_____ I cough or wheeze or my eyes water when I do laundry.
_____ I have other concerns. _____

_____

_____

_____

_____

_____

Do

_____ If you smell sewer gas in the room

        _____ Very gently, try to move the toilet. If the base moves even slightly in any direction, sewer gas may be escaping around the wax seal.

            _____ Have a plumber replace the seal.

_____ If a plumbing fixture has not been used for a while, pour a cup of water down the drain in the sink, tub, stall shower, or floor drain. (Sewer gas can leak up through a dried-out trap below the drain.)

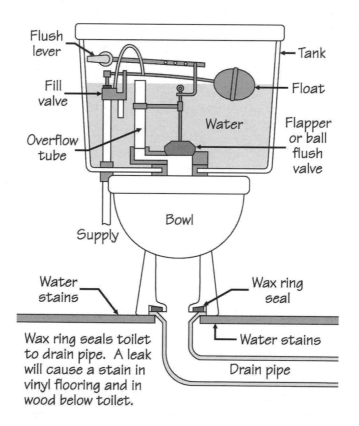

Flush lever · Tank · Fill valve · Float · Overflow tube · Water · Flapper or ball flush valve · Supply · Bowl · Water stains · Wax ring seal · Water stains · Drain pipe

Wax ring seals toilet to drain pipe. A leak will cause a stain in vinyl flooring and in wood below toilet.

If a toilet remains loose long enough, the floor around it may rot or even sprout mushrooms. Occasionally, a toilet with a broken seal will be secure yet still be the source of a sewer odor. *Tom Feiza, Mr. Fix-It, Inc.*

_____ Be sure the bathroom has adequate ventilation with an operable window and/or exhaust fan.

_____ If there is a urine smell in a bathroom, damp mop the floor and treat the baseboard convector near the toilet with steam vapor. (See Part I, Dilemma 1A, "My Basement.")

_____ Ventilate a bathroom well when using powerful cleaners.

_____ To minimize bioaerosol (airborne particulate matter from living things, such as bacteria), close the toilet lid before flushing.

Don't

_____ Leave strong cleaning compounds in a toilet for more than a few minutes. (Read manufacturer's cautions.)

_____ Burn scented jar candles in a bathroom. (They will stain the ceiling with soot.)

➤ The Kitchen

Do

_____ Have a technician

      _____ Use a TIF 8800 or another kind of combustible gas detector to check for leaks in a gas stove.

      _____ Adjust the air vent or gas if a burner flame is yellow rather than blue. (See Part II, Dilemma 3C, "Smoke and Harmful Gases.")

_____ Be sure the ignition is on when you turn on a pilotless gas-stove burner.

_____ Be sure pilot lights haven't gone out on an older gas stove.

_____ Keep a carbon monoxide detector in your kitchen if you have a gas oven.

_____ Have an adequate exhaust — one that vents to the exterior — over the stove.

_____ Turn the exhaust fan on when cooking.

_____ Turn the exhaust fan on and open windows when operating any oven on "self-clean" cycle, because the process forms carbon monoxide.

_____ Soak smelly sponges either in an ammonia solution (approximately a quarter of a cup of ammonia to a cup of water) or in a dishwasher-detergent solution (a teaspoon of dishwashing liquid or powder in a cup of very hot water).

———— Or run the sponge along with your dishes through a dishwasher cycle.

———— Use a steam vapor machine instead of chemical cleaners to remove burned-on glaze in ovens and on pots. (See Part I, Dilemma 1A, "My Basement.")

Don't

———— Use flammable liquids around any appliance with a flame, including a pilot light, or around any electric appliance with a motor.

———— Use your gas stove for heating the house.

———— Use a gas-fired grill or charcoal barbecue

———— Inside the house, because the barbecue produces large amounts of carbon monoxide.

———— At the exterior near combustible siding.

———— On a wood deck attached to the house.

➤ Laundry Areas

Do

———— Use liquid detergents instead of powders; liquids don't produce irritating dust.

———— Clean up laundry detergent spills.

———— Have a professional periodically check the dryer hose for lint clogging.

———— Have the hose cleaned or replaced as needed.

———— Check behind the dryer every few weeks to be sure the hose isn't kinked or disconnected.

———— If your hose is disconnected, have it reconnected.

———— If your hose kinks, install a rectangular metal dryer hose adaptor with a tight, right-angle fitting at the bottom of the duct and a straight round fitting at the top (called a close-clearance dryer-vent periscope pipe). These ducts are available at many building supply stores and online. (See www.savemoneywithus.com/dryerproducts.html.)

_____ Inspect the combustion chamber in a gas dryer annually and remove the dust and lint as needed.

_____ If you have a clothes dryer in a mechanical closet that contains a gas-fired hot-water heater or furnace, have a louver door installed to the closet to avoid backdrafting of combustion products, including carbon monoxide, emitted by these pieces of mechanical equipment.

Don't

_____ Vent a dryer (especially a gas dryer) to the interior.

_____ Allow dust and lint to accumulate behind, under, or within the machine.

_____ Install your dryer in a location that requires a long dryer vent hose to reach the exterior. (A 25-foot run is considered too long by most manufacturers; refer to the manufacturer's directions and see www.naturalhandyman.com/iip/infxtra/infdry.html.)

➤ Indoor Pools and Hot Tubs

Do

_____ Periodically disinfect an indoor hot tub or pool cover.

_____ Keep an indoor hot tub or pool cover as dust-free as possible.

_____ Store pool chemicals safely and away from the house.

Don't

_____ Allow concentrated dry and/or liquid pool chemicals to mix.

➤ For People with Allergies, Asthma, or Environmental Sensitivities

Do

_____ If you are chemically sensitive, hang new vinyl items such as shower curtains outdoors to air out until the smell dissipates.

_____ If you use a commercial laundromat, hang your clothes to dry at home rather than using commercial dryers, which can contain residual chemicals from someone else's fabric softener sheet.

_____ Air out clothing that has been dry-cleaned before hanging it in your closet.

Don't

_____ Use fabric softeners in the washing machine or fabric softener sheets in the dryer.

_____ Use detergents that contain enzymes or fragrance.

_____ Hang clothes to dry outside during pollen season if you are allergic to pollen.

_____ Use spray air fresheners or plug-in fragrance emitters to mask odors.

CONNIE'S COMMENTS

After our first child, Ben, was born, Jeff began to cough all the time and get respiratory infections, and every morning he woke up with swollen eyes. After a few months his symptoms subsided. I figured he was just plagued with seasonal allergies, since Ben was born in the spring. (Jeff is allergic to pollen.) When our second child, Jessie, was born, Jeff had the same symptoms, and again I figured it was seasonal allergies because Jessie was born in the fall. (Jeff is also allergic to mold growing on fallen leaves.)

But I was wrong. When our children were infants, I added liquid fabric softener to the wash to make their clothing soft and fragrant. I often washed their clothing with some of our clothes and bedding. Jeff is sensitive to the chemicals in fabric softeners. I stopped using fabric softener, and Jeff's symptoms went away.

My Notes _____

_____

_____

_____

REMINDERS

1. *Vent bathrooms, stoves, and dryers to the exterior.*
2. *If the bathroom is clean and well-ventilated, the use of fragrances to mask odors should not be necessary.*

WARNING

Sewer gas can escape into a room through a loose toilet seal or a dried-out plumbing trap.

RELEVANT RESOURCES

Products

Combustible gas detector: Professional Equipment, Janesville, WI (800-334-9291, www.professionalequipment.com).

Dryer duct supplies: www.savemoneywithus.com/dryerproducts.html for close-clearance dryer-vent periscope pipes.

A Website

www.naturalhandyman.com/iip/infxtra/infdry/html: For information about optimum length of dryer exhaust hoses.

B. OTHER ROOMS AND THEIR CONTENTS

_____ I have increased asthma or allergy symptoms when in bed or first thing in the morning.

_____ I cough, my eyes water, or I get headaches or other health symptoms after spending time in a carpeted space.

_____ A new carpet smells terrible.

_____ New furniture has an irritating smell.

_____ I get headaches when I'm around a copier or printer.

_____ I have other concerns. _____

_____

_____

JEFF'S GEMS

Mattresses and pillows can be infested with dust mites. Furniture, office equipment, and new carpeting can off-gas (emit) irritating chemicals. Rugs can contain animal dander that becomes airborne with foot traffic. Wool rugs can shed microscopic wool-fiber fragments that can be irritating. Feather quilts, pillows, and cushions can emit legions of respirable, irritating particles.

CONNIE'S COMMENTS

All true, but he is really a "cup half empty" kind of guy, isn't he?

➤ Beds and Bedding

Do

_____ Wash sheets weekly in hot water (130°F).

_____ Wash and thoroughly dry mattress pads every other week.

_____ Wash blankets monthly.

_____ Tumble blankets and quilts in a dryer on a low to medium setting for 10 minutes once a week.

_____ Place stuffed animals you keep on the bed in a dryer on low for 10 minutes once a week.

CONNIE'S COMMENTS

Be careful not to melt anything in the dryer, like those fuzzy blankets — the kind they have in hotels — or a much-beloved stuffed animal, by using too high a setting or leaving the object in the dryer too long.

Don't

_____ Overload beds with pillows or stuffed animals.

_____ Wash stuffed animals. (They often remain damp long enough to host microbial growth.)

_____ Use secondhand mattresses, even if they are gifts from family or friends, because you never know what might be lurking within.

JEFF'S GEMS

We spend up to a third of our day in bed, and as we move around in our sleep, dust mite fecal pellets and body parts as well as feather fragments from down pillows or quilts can become airborne and may be inhaled. When you acquire a used mattress, it may already be contaminated with these allergens.

CONNIE'S COMMENTS

Not a pretty picture, is it?

➤ Carpeting

Do

_____ If a strong odor appears after a new wall-to-wall carpet or rug is installed, the area should be well ventilated until the odor disappears.

    _____ The carpet as well as pad beneath it may have to be replaced if the odor persists for more than a month.

_____ Hire professionals trained by the Institute of Inspection, Cleaning, and Restoration Certification (IICRC) to clean wall-to-wall carpeting.

_____ Use steam vapor to kill fleas, booklice, silverfish, spiders, and mites. (See Part I, Dilemma 1A, "My Basement.")

    _____ Spot check some of the carpet first to be sure that the steam won't damage the fibers.

    _____ Follow the manufacturer's directions for safe use of the machine.

_____ If you think a carpet may be contaminated with lead dust, take a vacuum sample and have it tested by a lab.

    _____ If the carpet is contaminated, professionals should remove the carpet under containment. (See Part I, Dilemma 1A, "My Basement.")

_____ Send rugs out periodically for professional cleaning.

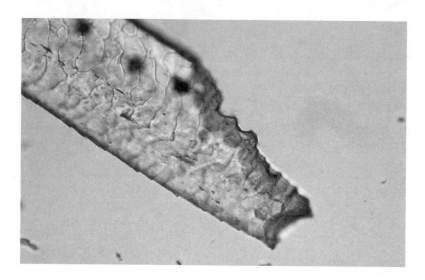

Carpet beetles are small enough to be missed but still big enough to see: about 1/8 inch long. Carpet beetle larvae feed on wool fibers, like the one in this photomicrograph. You can see individual bites at one end of the wool fiber. *May Indoor Air Investigations LLC*

Don't
_____ Wash your own carpets.
_____ Have carpets washed during humid weather.

➤ Furniture

Do
_____ If new furniture emits an odor, ventilate the space for several days.
　　　_____ If the odor persists for more than a few months, the furniture may have to be replaced.
_____ If you wonder whether new furniture is off-gassing, use the paper-towel test. (See Part I, Dilemma 1H, "Hotels and Automobiles.")
_____ If you suspect that an item in the room is off-gassing, either remove the item or, if it is too large to move, wrap it in aluminum foil.
_____ If you can't find the source of an odor, remove all the furnishings in a room and then reintroduce them one by one to see if the smell returns.

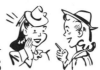

OTHER VOICES: CASE STUDIES

New products can be a problem. One client ordered a custom-made, feather-filled couch for which she paid over $3,000. She could not sit on it without experiencing allergy symptoms and a headache, but the company that made the couch wouldn't take it back or refund her money. The woman asked me if I could figure out why the couch was bothering her. I took a dust sample from the cushions and discovered several different types of feathers as well as many dust-mite droppings. The only way this could have happened was if the couch had been made from "recycled" feathers! The woman used my report to get her refund.

Another client had a child who had been experiencing asthma symptoms ever since he started sleeping on his expensive new mattress. The department store insisted that there was no problem with the mattress, but I took a dust sample from it and found pollen, mold spores, and wood char. The pollen and mold spores were signs that the mattress had been outdoors — rather unusual for a new mattress! I think the presence of wood char suggested that the "new" mattress had been in a warehouse fire, and perhaps then cleaned and set outdoors to dry.

► Home Office Equipment

Do

_____ Place a printer or copier in a space with adequate ventilation.
_____ Return a monitor or printer that off-gasses a strong chemical odor for more than three days.

► For People with Allergies, Asthma, or Environmental Sensitivities

Do

_____ Use allergen-control encasings on *all* pillows and mattresses, including sofa beds, rather than just on the pillows and mattresses belonging to family members with allergies or asthma.
_____ Use only dust-mite control encasings backed with a solid-plastic

What and Where?   123

film like polyurethane. (Try cotton knit or tricot knit; see www
.onlineallergyrelief.com or www.allergycontrolproducts.com.)

_____ Put two encasings on a mattress if one must be removed
periodically for cleaning.

_____ Put an allergen-control encasing on an older box spring.

_____ Vacuum cushioned items with a HEPA vacuum (a vacuum with high
efficiency particulate arrestance filtration).

_____ Tumble your pillows every week in the dryer on low for 10 minutes
and replace them once a year if you don't have them covered with
allergen-control encasings.

_____ Ask a hotel for foam- or polyester-filled pillows (or pillows filled with
some other synthetic material or with cotton) as well as polyester- or
cotton-filled quilts if feathers bother you.

_____ Sniff-test a carpet sample before installing new wall-to-wall carpeting
to see if it emits a smell you find irritating.

_____ Sniff-test a carpet pad before buying it. (You may have to make an
opening in the plastic wrapper.)

_____ Ask the manufacturer for specific information about a carpet's or
pad's emissions.

_____ Use a leather-covered rather than fabric-covered desk chair, which
can become infested with mites if used frequently and for long
periods of time.

_____ Use leather or futon couches rather than upholstered couches.

_____ Cover the mattresses on futon couches with allergen-control
encasings.

_____ If you are sensitive to formaldehyde

_____ Seal exposed edges and plug unused shelf holes in laminate
cabinets.

_____ Seal all bare particle-board surfaces with an acceptable finish
(such as an AFM — American Formulating and Manufacturing — product) or with diluted Elmer's glue (one part
glue to one or two parts water).

_____ Check that varnish on furniture doesn't contain urea
formaldehyde.

_____ Avoid owning furniture with particle board made with urea-
formaldehyde glue.

Don't

_____ Use down pillows and quilts.

_____ Remove allergen-control encasings from mattresses or pillows, because this releases allergens.

_____ Vacuum older mattresses, especially if they are not encased in allergen-control covers or if you don't have a HEPA vacuum.

_____ Use wool blankets if you are sensitive to wool.

_____ Use fragranced products to clean carpets.

_____ Install carpeting with styrene-butadiene (latex) backing or with adhesives with high emission rates of volatile organic compounds (VOCs). Manufacturer's specs can tell you about the emission rates of carpeting you are considering purchasing.

_____ Buy a carpet with an odor you find irritating.

_____ Buy a carpet backed with or a carpet pad made out of material that emits a rubber-like odor.

_____ Buy furniture with urea-formaldehyde varnish or furniture made from medium-density fiber or particle board if you are sensitive to formaldehyde.

_____ Leave stairway carpets in place when you move into an older home.

OTHER VOICES: Q & A

Q: Ever since we installed a new carpet there has been a strong smell in the room, and I get a headache every time I spend extended time there. Could the new carpet be causing my symptoms?

A: Yes, in a word. Some people are sensitized already to the chemicals that off-gas from new carpets, while other people develop a hypersensitivity to these chemicals after being exposed. That "new carpet odor" is caused by the emission of vapors from the adhesive used to attach the fibers to the backing. Carpet manufacturers recommend that spaces with new carpeting be ventilated with lots of fresh air for a few days prior to occupancy, but sometimes new carpets continue to off-gas for many months.

Ventilate the room and avoid spending time there for a few days. If your symptoms persist, you may have to get rid of the carpet.

Q: I bought a new set of book shelves for my living room and I swear that every time I sit in the room, I sense a funny, irritating smell. Am I crazy?

A: If the shelves are made of medium-density fiberboard or particle board, the material may be off-gassing formaldehyde, which can irritate mucous membranes. Formaldehyde is not emitted from the laminated surfaces. Most of the chemical off-gases from unfinished surfaces, like exposed peg holes and shelf edges and bottoms. The odor may dissipate in a matter of weeks or months, but sometimes furniture like this will continue to off-gas for over a year.

You can buy a passive test kit for formaldehyde (usually available at labs for under $100). You can also remove the shelves and see if you feel better in the room. If you can't remove or return the shelving, try sealing all the exposed particle board surfaces with two coats of varnish. If you are chemically sensitive and you find the smell of varnish irritating, you can try to seal the unfinished surfaces with a solution of Elmer's glue (approximately one to two parts water to one part glue). Livos also makes paint for people with chemical sensitivities (www.livos.com).

My Notes _____

_____

_____

_____

_____

_____

_____

_____

REMINDERS

1. *If you or anyone in your family is allergic to dust mites, cover all mattresses and pillows with allergen-control encasings.*
2. *Research carpeting before you have it installed to find out about its chemical emissions.*

Some printers and copiers emit potentially irritating chemicals when in use, though the amount will depend on relative humidity and extent of use.

RELEVANT RESOURCES

Laboratories That Sell Test Kits and Analyze Dust Samples from Carpeting and Rugs

Aerotech Labs, Phoenix, AZ (800-651-4802, www.aerotechpk.com).

DACI Laboratory, Johns Hopkins University Asthma and Allergy Center, Baltimore, MD (800-344-3224, www.hopkinsmedicine.org/allergy/daci/index.html).

Envirologix, Portland, ME (866-408-4597, http://envirologix.com).

Northeast Laboratory, Winslow, ME (800-244-8378, www.nelabservices.com).

Organizations

Institute of Inspection, Cleaning, and Restoration Certification (IICRC), Vancouver, WA (800-835-4624, www.certifiedcleaners.org).

Restoration Industry Association (RIA), Columbia, MD (800 272 7012, www.ascr.org).

Products

Allergen-control covers for mattresses and pillows: cotton knit or tricot knit covers with solid-plastic film (like polyurethane) under cotton are best. (See www.onlineallergyrelief.com or www.allergycontrolproducts.com.)

Carpet covering (self-adhering clear plastic): Pro-Tect Associates, Inc., Northfield, IL (800-545-0826, www.pro-tect.com).

Dennyfoil: a paper-aluminum foil laminate that can be used to temporarily cover surfaces that emit odors. Denny Wholesale, Boca Raton, FL (561-750-3705, www.dennywholesale.com).

Dust mite allergen test kit: DACI Laboratory, Johns Hopkins University Asthma and Allergy Center, Baltimore, MD (800-344-3224, www.hopkinsmedicine.org/allergy/daci/index.html).

Formaldehyde test kit: SKC Inc., Eighty Four, PA (800-752-8472, www.skcinc.com).

HEPA vacuum: Available in retail vacuum and home supply stores, as well as online. (See www.miele.com.)

Paint for people with chemical sensitivities: Livos, Pine Plains, NY (800-343-6394, www.livos.com); AFM products (800-239-0321; www.afmsafecoat.com).

A Publication

The Healthy House, John Bower. Bloomington, IN: Healthy House Institute, 2001.

C. SMOKE AND HARMFUL GASES

_____ I can smell smoke from someone else's fireplace or wood stove.

_____ Smoke comes out of my fireplace or wood stove into the room.

_____ I get headaches when my gas fireplace is running.

_____ I live above someone who smokes, and the cigarette smoke is entering my apartment.

_____ I can smell gasoline from the garage next to or underneath where I live.

_____ I'm worried about radon in my house.

_____ I have other concerns. _____

_____

_____

➤ Fireplaces, Wood Stoves, and Cigarettes

JEFF'S GEMS

There's little you can do to avoid smelling wood smoke from nearby chimneys, other than ask your neighbor to refrain from using his or her fireplace or wood stove. Installing tight windows may also help reduce the amount of smoke infiltrating your house. But during the heating season, warm buoyant air inevitably leaks out of the upper floors of a house, and outdoor air flows into the house to replace the lost air. Thus, whatever odor is outdoors finds its way indoors.

If you have a fireplace or wood stove in your home, tend the fire carefully; otherwise, the flames may produce irritating and even toxic combustion products or could spread, causing destruction to the building.

Do

_____ Check to be sure the damper is open before lighting a fire.

    _____ Be sure the fireplace damper or wood stove doors are closed when the fireplace or stove is not in use, particularly if you have an exterior chimney.

    _____ Be sure the ashes are completely cold before fully closing the damper.

    _____ If concerned about heat loss, have fireplace doors installed.

JEFF'S GEMS

By heat loss, I don't mean losing heat from the fire. I mean losing heat because house air goes up the chimney along with the smoke, drawing warm air from other areas of the house into the room where the fireplace is located. If you install fireplace doors, you reduce that air flow while still leaving enough draft for the fire.

_____ Use only properly dried wood or fire logs.

_____ Have your flues inspected regularly and cleaned as needed, to improve the draft and avoid creosote buildup in your chimney that can lead to a chimney fire.

_____ If you are living in a new, fairly airtight house, be sure the fireplace has its own source of combustion air; otherwise, backdrafting of combustion products (including carbon monoxide) can occur.

_____ If you are using a gas fireplace that vents to the interior and there is condensation on the windows when the fireplace is running, try using the fireplace less frequently.

_____ If your gas fireplace exhausts to the exterior and there is condensation on the windows when the fireplace is running, stop using the fireplace, open a window to introduce fresh air into the space, and call a technician to make repairs.

JEFF'S GEMS

Combustion of gas produces water vapor. If you see condensation on your windows when your gas fireplace is running, it may mean that combustion products are entering the room, perhaps because the fireplace exhausts to the interior. Even if the fireplace exhausts to the exterior, there may be insufficient draft due to wind conditions outside or blockage in the vent pipe, or the house may be overly airtight. If a house is very airtight, opening a window slightly may provide enough air to reverse a backdraft.

A great tool for testing draft and air flows is a Wizard Stick. (See www .zerotoys.com.) This children's toy produces safe smoke that can be used to trace all sorts of air flows, including draft and exhaust (from a kitchen or bathroom fan, for example).

_____ Keep a carbon monoxide detector and a five-pound dry powder fire extinguisher in the room where your gas or wood fireplace or stove is located.

_____ Advocate for a cigarette smoke–free indoor environment.

Don't
_____ Put ashes into a combustible receptacle or in a metal container without legs.

_____ Put ashes in a dumpster or on a wood deck.

_____ Shut down a wood stove too tightly at night, because the draft may reverse and combustion products, including carbon monoxide, may flow into the room.

_____ Shut down a wood stove or close a fireplace damper until the ashes have been cooling for at least 24 hours. (Embers in ashes can burn for days.)

_____ Leave a fire in a wood stove or fireplace unattended.
_____ Use fluid to start a fire.
_____ Allow smoking indoors.

OTHER VOICES: Q & A

Q: *I work in a room on the second floor of a Victorian single family that has been converted to office space. Someone who works on the first floor is allowed to smoke in his office. The smell of cigarette smoke drifts up into my office and makes me feel sick. Is there anything I can do to prevent the smell from entering my office?*

A: *It's difficult to prevent cigarette smoke from being carried on air flows into other parts of a building. The best thing you can do is try to have cigarette smoking banned inside the building. In the end, though, you may have to ask to be relocated or find another job in a building in which smoking is not allowed.*

JEFF'S GEMS

Secondhand smoke can be irritating, can exacerbate asthma symptoms, and can even be carcinogenic, so smoking should not be allowed in public buildings or near the entranceways to such buildings. In my opinion, smoking should be banned in all buildings, whether public or private, and whether manufacturing, industrial, office, or residential.

► Gases

Do
_____ Keep a door leading from a garage into habitable space airtight (gasketed) and closed.
_____ Seal pipe openings in walls, ceilings, or floors in a building with an underground garage.

———— Whenever possible, store fuel as well as gasoline-powered equipment in a detached shed or garage.

———— Buy a radon test kit if you are worried about levels of radon in air in your home or below-grade (partially or fully below ground level) office. (See Part II, Dilemma 5, "Testing.")

JEFF'S GEMS

Radon in the air is odorless and colorless, and while it does not have immediate effects on human health, it can cause lung cancer after years of exposure.

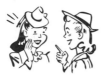

OTHER VOICES: Q & A

Q: Should I avoid living in a house with a radon mitigation system?

A: Sometimes such systems are installed in new homes as a caution, even if radon levels are not excessive. If radon levels are high, a sub-slab depressurization radon mitigation system is a very effective remediation tool if installed properly. There is also some evidence that a radon mitigation system reduces the water vapor infiltration through the basement floor and foundation walls.

Occasionally, such systems are installed to remediate other soil gas problems, such as chemical fumes arising from spills into the soil, or even from a nearby residential or commercial buried tank leaking fuel or other chemicals. If the radon system was installed to remediate a volatile organic compound problem like this, I recommend you research the history of the problem very carefully so that you can make an informed decision. If there is a small amount of some chemical in the soil and the radon mitigation system solves the problem, that's probably acceptable (unless someone in your family is chemically sensitive). On the other hand, if there is some unknown amount of solvent or fuel leaking from a nearby source, I'd think twice about living there.

Don't

_____ Use solvents indoors unless there is plenty of ventilation.

_____ Let a car idle in an attached garage, even if the garage door is open.

_____ Automatically blame radon in air for symptoms you experience when you are in a building. Instead, confer with an IAQ professional to find out what conditions in your building may be leading to your symptoms and see your physician.

▶ For People with Allergies, Asthma, or Environmental Sensitivities

Do

_____ If someone you live or work with wears heavily fragranced shampoo, deodorant, perfume, or cologne that irritates you, ask the person to stop using that product and find an unscented alternative.

_____ Advocate to have smoking banned near entrances to and exits from your building.

Don't

_____ Use a gas fireplace that vents combustion gases to the interior.

_____ Burn poison ivy or oak; people who are sensitized can react even to the smoke.

_____ Store gasoline-powered equipment that may leak (like lawn mowers) in a basement or a garage attached to or underneath habitable space.

_____ Wear heavily fragranced personal products.

_____ Use plug-in fragrance emitters.

_____ Burn fragranced candles if you or someone you live with finds the scent irritating.

_____ Burn jar candles.

My Notes _____

_____

_____

_____

_____

_____

_____

_____

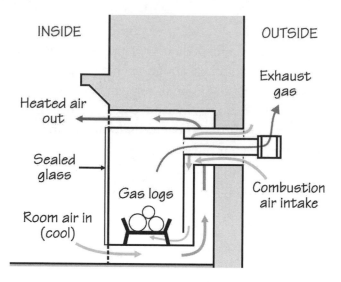

If a strong wind blows against the vent pipe of a direct-vent fireplace, backdrafting can occur. The illustration shows how some fireplaces heat room air by circulating it around the hot fire box. *Tom Feiza, Mr. Fix-It, Inc.*

REMINDERS

1. *Have your chimney inspected yearly and cleaned as needed.*
2. *Don't use solvents indoors unless there is plenty of ventilation.*
3. *Be sure you know why a radon system was installed in a property.*
4. *Test any below-grade spaces where you live or work for radon in air.*

WARNINGS

1. *Ashes that seem cold can still contain burning embers hot enough to start a fire.*
2. *Chimney fires are caused by a buildup of creosote in the chimney.*
3. *Gas fireplaces can produce carbon monoxide.*
4. *Secondhand cigarette smoke can be carcinogenic.*

5. *Fragrances are chemicals and can be irritating to those who are sensitized or have asthma.*

CONNIE'S COMMENTS

I used to smoke. Well, that's an understatement. I used to smoke a lot. When Jeff and I were first dating he had quit smoking but was beginning to pick up the habit again because he was spending time with me. He asked me to quit, and I was pretty interested in him, so I complied. That was 31 years ago, and I still feel a weak craving now and then when I'm sitting next to someone who's smoking. I guess that's why they call smoking an addiction. Good thing I quit. I'd probably have developed lung cancer by now if I hadn't.

RELEVANT RESOURCES

Products

A radon test kit generally costs less than $40 and is available in many hardware and building supply stores.

Wizard Stick, useful for tracking airflows through your home: Available through Zero Toys, Concord, MA (978-371-3378, www.zerotoys.com).

Publications

"A Citizen's Guide to Radon," an EPA publication available through the Indoor Air Quality Information Clearing House (800-438-4318, www.epa.gov/iaq).

The Healthy House, John Bower. Bloomington, IN: Healthy House Institute, 2001.

Radon-Specific Publications and Resources, Environmental Protection Agency, Washington, DC (www.epa.gov/radon/pubs).

D. HEATING AND COOLING SYSTEMS

_____ I or someone in my family gets a headache sometimes when the heat is on.
_____ The air seems stuffy.
_____ There's a thumping noise when the furnace or air conditioning system turns on or off.

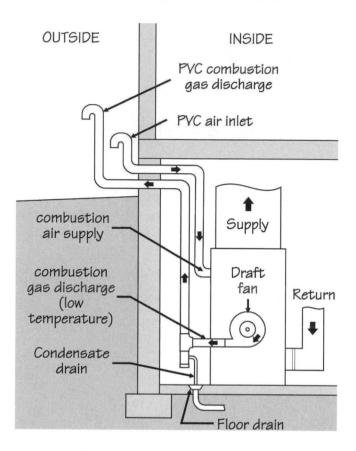

OUTSIDE   INSIDE

PVC combustion
gas discharge

PVC air inlet

combustion
air supply

Supply

combustion
gas discharge
(low
temperature)

Draft
fan

Return

Condensate
drain

Floor drain

In the winter you can easily spot a home with a direct-vent furnace or boiler because steam is blowing out of a plastic or metal pipe near the foundation. There are usually two pipes: one to suck in air for combustion (combustion air) and one to exhaust the combustion products. Sometimes, the two pipes are "concentric" (one is inside the other), and only the discharge vent is obvious. *Tom Feiza, Mr. Fix-It, Inc.*

_____ I can sense a vibration when the furnace or air conditioning system
turns on or off.
_____ In the heating season, some rooms seem chilly.
_____ In the cooling season, some rooms seem too warm.
_____ There's a gas or oil smell near the furnace or boiler.
_____ I have other concerns. _____
_____
_____
_____

Questions to Answer

1. How is your heat supplied — by forced air, by water in radiators or base-board convectors, or by steam in radiators? _____
2. Where is your boiler or furnace? _____
   (A boiler heats water for radiators or baseboard convectors, or steam for radiators. A furnace heats air, not water.)
3. Is it direct-vented? _____
   (A direct-vent boiler or furnace vents to the exterior, often at a side wall through metal or plastic piping, rather than into a chimney.)
4. Do you have a hydro-air system? _____
   (A hydro-air system has a boiler to heat water, which is piped to two or more remote air-handling units, or AHUs, with heating coils.)
5. If you have a heat pump, where is the indoor unit located? _____
   (A heat pump is a split system with an indoor unit and an outdoor unit. The blower and heat exchange coil, together called the air-handling unit, are indoors, and the compressor is outdoors.)

_____

JEFF'S GEMS

When I ask clients about their heating or cooling system, more often than not I am greeted with blank stares. The only component that people are often familiar with is the thermostat.

The questions above aren't all directly connected to indoor air quality, but please take some time to try to answer them nonetheless. Have a knowledge-able friend, HVAC (heating, ventilation, and air conditioning) technician, or home inspector explain the basic components of your heating or cooling system to you. In the end, you should know what type of system you have and where the system's components are located, among other practical details of the workings of the system. Then you can ask questions relevant to your indoor air quality concerns, as well as be more knowledgeable when your mechanical system develops problems.

➤ Air Conveyance Systems

Do

_____ If the ducts make noise when the blower turns on and off, check to be sure the returns aren't covered with rugs or furniture.

     _____ If the returns aren't blocked, have an HVAC technician check the system.

_____ If the furnace or air conditioner vibrates, have a professional check to see if the blower is dirty or unbalanced.

_____ If some rooms are too cool in the heating season or too warm in the cooling season, check your ductwork for kinks, blockage, or loose connections.

     _____ Have an HVAC (heating, ventilation, and air conditioning) technician check to see that your system is balanced and has an adequate number of supplies and returns, and that flexible supply ducts aren't so long that air flow is reduced.

Don't

_____ Block return grilles with rugs or furniture.

➤ Gas-Fired Equipment

Do

_____ Vent a gas clothes dryer to the exterior, rather than into a basement, garage, or habitable space.

_____ Have carbon monoxide detectors near bedrooms and heating equipment and in rooms next to or above garages.

_____ Have a kill switch installed in the attic for a whole-house fan to prevent accidental winter operation when windows are closed; otherwise, combustion products including carbon monoxide may backdraft into habitable spaces.

_____ Check the condition of the vent pipe for a boiler, furnace, or hot-water heater.

     _____ If the piping is metal, the sections should all be screwed together (three screws per connection).

     _____ There should be no rusted pin holes in the piping.

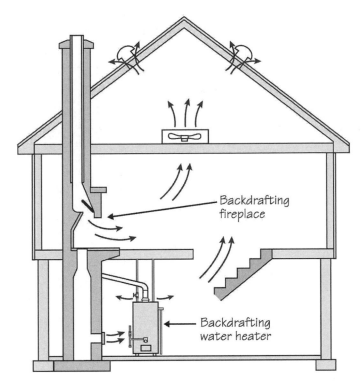

Whole house fans can cause serious negative pressure in a home if windows are not open. Fireplaces and gas-fired appliances can backdraft.

Whole-house fans are great for summer use to cool a house but they must be used with caution. *Tom Feiza, Mr. Fix-It, Inc.*

_____ The end of the pipe should be securely inserted into the chimney.
_____ All the access panels to a furnace, boiler, or hot-water heater should be securely in place.

CONNIE'S COMMENTS

When Jeff and I were first married, I used to sell real estate part time. Once when I was running a Sunday open house at a property that was unoccupied, I was alone in the kitchen, waiting for people to show up. Suddenly I felt dizzy and disoriented. I opened several windows in the house, ran outside to the yard, and used my cell phone to call the gas company. I found out afterward that there was a hole in the chimney in the family room next to the kitchen, and combustion products were pouring into the room. Luckily I left before succumbing to carbon monoxide poisoning, but it was a pretty scary experience. It also marked the beginning of the end of my real estate career.

_____ If your gas boiler or furnace is direct-vented

    _____ Check pipes periodically to see that they are securely connected to each other.

    _____ In winter, check that the end of the exhaust pipe is not blocked by snow or ice.

    _____ Have a technician raise an exhaust pipe that gets buried by snow.

JEFF'S GEMS

For centuries, hot, toxic combustion products like smoke went up chimneys and into the air, where they usually rose up and away from the building. This certainly made sense, but unfortunately, about one quarter to one half of the available energy from the fuel also went up the chimney and was wasted. Since the energy crisis of the 1970s, engineers have been designing combustion appliances like furnaces, boilers, and water heaters to be ever more efficient.

Today, more heat is taken out of combustion products before they leave the appliance. This means cooler exhaust gases and smaller volumes of them. These gases can no longer be vented through a big masonry chimney, because they aren't hot enough to create enough draft. Direct venting was developed to solve this problem.

In direct venting, combustion gases go through plastic or metal piping and usually exit the house from a side wall rather than above the roof. The oxygen needed for combustion usually comes from a second plastic pipe open to the air at the side wall of the house and connected directly to the combustion appliance.

One problem with direct venting is that toxic gases are now discharged at the side of the house rather than above the roof. When warm toxic gases rise from a side-wall vent, they sometimes get drawn back into the house by infiltration through construction gaps or open windows. Sensitized individuals may be affected by the odor or gases.

_____ Check the flame on your furnace or boiler to be sure it's blue rather than yellow. (Though oil flames are supposed to be yellow, a yellow flame on a gas-fired boiler or furnace may be producing carbon monoxide.)

    _____ Call a technician if necessary to check the furnace or boiler.

_____ Have an HVAC (heating, ventilation, and air conditioning) technician

    _____ Check the condition of the exterior of your boiler.

    _____ Check the burners and interior of the combustion chamber to be sure all is clean.

    _____ Check the exterior of mechanical equipment (boiler, furnace, hot-water heater) with a mirror or a combustible gas detector to be sure combustion products are going into the chimney rather than leaking out into the mechanical room or basement.

_____ If you find any new soot or scorch marks, corrosion, or burned paint on the outside of your boiler

    _____ Turn down your thermostat.

    _____ If weather permits, turn your furnace or boiler off.

    _____ Open your windows

    _____ Call your heating company immediately for service.

        _____ Have the technician check for combustion spillage.

_____ If you find any new soot or scorch marks, corrosion, or burned paint on the outside of your hot-water heater, have a technician check the appliance for combustion spillage.

► Oil-Fired Equipment

Do

_____ Have carbon monoxide detectors near bedrooms and heating equipment.

_____ Have a kill switch installed in the attic for a whole-house fan to prevent accidental winter operation when windows are closed; otherwise, combustion products may backdraft into habitable spaces, causing a puff-back that may blacken the interior of your home.

_____ Check the condition of the vent pipe for a boiler, furnace, or hot-water heater.

    _____ If the piping is metal, the sections should all be screwed together (three screws per connection).

    _____ There should be no rusted pin holes in the piping.

    _____ All the access panels to the furnace, boiler, or hot-water heater should be securely in place.

    _____ The end of the pipe should be securely inserted into the chimney.

_____ Be certain that the interior of your boiler is brush-cleaned at least every other year.

JEFF'S GEMS

All oil companies provide a yearly maintenance service to their customers, because unlike gas flames, oil flames can produce soot and other solid particles that can build up in and block combustion-gas pathways. This yearly tune-up usually involves cleaning or replacing the burner nozzle, but at least every other year should also include a thorough brush-cleaning of the boiler interior. When an oil-service company says that it has "cleaned" your boiler, this often only means that the burner nozzle has been cleaned.

It's not uncommon to find the interior of an oil burner clogged with debris if it has not been brush-cleaned often enough. Occasionally the boiler interior is so clogged that soot and combustion products go into the house, rather than going up the chimney, and cause a "puff-back." A puff-back makes the house smell like oil and soot, stains surfaces black, and can result in thousands of dollars spent cleaning up the mess.

If your oil technician spends less than half an hour on your annual tune-up, you may be headed for a puff-back. To brush-clean a boiler interior, part of the outside metal case often must be removed. The entire cleaning process can take two to three hours to complete.

_____ If your boiler is direct-vented

      _____ Check pipes periodically to see that they are securely connected to each other.

      _____ In winter, check that the end of the exhaust pipe is not blocked by snow or ice.

      _____ Have a technician raise an exhaust pipe that gets buried by snow.

_____ If you are having headaches or get a funny taste in your mouth when the heat turns on

      _____ Turn down the thermostat.

      _____ If weather permits, turn the boiler off.

      _____ Open your windows.

      _____ Call your heating company for immediate service.

_____ Have an HVAC technician annually

      _____ Check the condition of the exterior of your boiler.

      _____ Check the interior of the combustion chamber to be sure all is clean.

      _____ Check oil lines for leaks.

      _____ Install an oil-safety valve on the oil tank.

      _____ Place the oil-supply line in a leaktight liner.

_____ Using a flashlight and mirror, check a basement oil tank for leaks, particularly at the oil filter and bottom of tank.

_____ Place a can or tray under an area of your basement oil tank that you suspect is leaking and check periodically for fluid.

      _____ Have any oil-line or fitting leak repaired.

      _____ Replace a tank that is leaking from a corroded bottom.

JEFF'S GEMS

Ultrasonic tank-testing can be used to assess the condition of an above-ground oil tank. Check your phone book or the Internet to find a company in your area that can provide this service.

———— Have professionals clean up a significant oil leak.

———— If you notice any new soot, corrosion, or scorch marks or burned paint on the outside of your boiler

    ———— Turn down your thermostat.

    ———— If weather permits, turn your furnace or boiler off.

    ———— Open your windows.

    ———— Call your heating company immediately for service.

        ———— Have the technician check for combustion spillage.

———— If you find any soot, corrosion, or scorch marks or burned paint on the outside of your hot-water heater, have a technician check the appliance for combustion spillage.

———— If you are switching to gas and are having the basement oil tank removed, have the oil-fill and vent pipes removed at the same time.

JEFF'S GEMS

If your heat was switched from oil to gas and a basement oil tank was removed from the property, check to be sure the fill pipe was also removed. If the pipe was left in place, oil-delivery personnel might show up at the wrong address and fill your basement with oil: an environmental disaster! This scenario may sound unlikely, but it happens at least once a year in the Boston area, where Connie and I live.

———— Check your local and state regulations regarding leak-testing and replacement requirements for a residential buried oil tank you are still using.

———— Have an abandoned buried oil tank professionally removed.

    ———— Confer with your local fire department about permits and regulations.

    ———— Be sure the contractor follows relevant local and state regulations.

Don't

_____ Delay having oil tanks or lines repaired.

_____ Repair rather than replace a corroded leaking oil tank.

_____ Leave the oil-fill pipe and vent pipe in place if your basement oil tank has been removed.

_____ Direct vent any oil-combustion equipment, because the oil odor inevitably enters the house.

➤ Fire

Don't

_____ Place any combustible materials near electric baseboard heaters, vent pipes, or metal surfaces that are in contact with hot combustion gases.

_____ Dry laundry on vent pipes from a boiler, furnace, or water heater.

_____ Place anything combustible within three feet of a boiler or hot-water heater.

_____ Let electric cords touch electric baseboard heaters.

➤ For People with Allergies, Asthma, or Environmental Sensitivities

Do

_____ Using a combustible gas detector like a TIFF 8800, periodically test all gas pipes, fittings, and gas-fired equipment for leaks.

Don't

_____ Allow an oil company technician to use fragranced masking powder when cleaning up a small oil leak.

My Notes _____

_____

_____

_____

_____

_____

_____

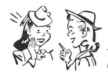

OTHER VOICES: Q & A

Q: I live in a townhouse, and my hot-air furnace is located in a small closet on the ground floor. When the heat is on I sometimes get headaches, mostly when I am upstairs in the living room, which is located above that closet. Could the heat be causing this problem?

A: You don't mention smelling oil. When an oil-fired furnace or boiler leaks combustion products, people also generally smell oil. I'm therefore assuming that you have a gas-fired furnace.

Your symptoms may be caused by combustion products that contain carbon monoxide. Combustion products can get into the air from the room housing your mechanical equipment or even from the duct system, if it contains holes or gaps. If combustion gases are being distributed by your duct system, you should experience symptoms in every room. Then the furnace heat exchanger will have to be checked immediately to see if it is cracked and allowing combustion products to leak into the air circulation.

Since you mention having particular trouble in the living room, though, I suspect that combustion products are leaking from the furnace into your mechanical closet as soon as the burner lights. Perhaps there is spillage from a disconnected vent pipe, gas pressure that is too high, dirty burners, or inadequate draft due to a blocked chimney. Combustion gases are hot, so they float to the ceiling and from there can flow up the stairway to the first floor and into your living room.

Turn your heat down as low as you can so that the furnace will not run as often, or if weather permits, turn the heat off completely. Open your windows and call a technician to come as soon as possible to check for combustion products leaking from the furnace, vent system, or heat exchanger. You should also have one carbon monoxide detector in the mechanical closet and another near the stairs leading up from the ground level.

REMINDER

Keep your mechanical equipment clean and in good working order.

WARNINGS

1. *Operating a whole-house fan without opening windows can result in backdrafting of combustion products into habitable spaces.*
2. *If the ducts are making a thumping noise or the furnace is vibrating, not only is the noise annoying, but potentially irritating particles within the system can be loosened and become aerosolized.*

RELEVANT RESOURCES

An Institute That Trains and Certifies HVAC Professionals

New England Fuel Institute (NEFI), Watertown, MA (617-924-1000; www.nefi.com).

Organizations

Air Conditioning Contractors of America, Arlington, VA (703-575-4477, www.acca.org).

Sheet Metal and Air Conditioning Contractors' National Association, Inc. (SMACNA), Chantilly, VA (703-803-2980, www.smacna.org).

Products

Carbon monoxide monitor: NSI 3000 low-level CO monitor from National Comfort Institute, Sheffield Lake, OH (800-633-7058, www.nationalcomfortinstitute .com).

Combustible gas detector: Professional Equipment, Janesville, WI (800-334-9291, www.professionalequipment.com).

E. PETS AND PESTS

_____ I have allergy or asthma symptoms when near certain pets or their owners.

_____ I think we have a mouse infestation.

_____ There's a terrible smell in one area of the building, and I wonder if it's caused by pests.

Where? _____

What is the smell like? _____

Is the smell there all the time or only sometimes? _____

If the smell is intermittent, when is it strongest? _____

_____ I think I have a cockroach infestation.

_____ I see moths in my house

      _____ In the kitchen.

      _____ In rooms with rugs.

      _____ In closets.

_____ I have other concerns. _____

_____

_____

_____

JEFF'S GEMS

Animals don't have to be present to cause problems for those with certain allergies. People who own cats, dogs, and other pets with hair or fur can have pet hair and dander on their clothing. In a Swedish study of 22 day care centers, cat and dog allergens were detected in all of the centers, even though pets weren't allowed in any of them. And pests such as cockroaches, mites, and flour or wool moths can also cause symptoms for those who are sensitized.

➤ Pets

Do

_____ Use a folded blanket that can be washed every other week for a pet bed, rather than a store-bought pet bed that cannot be washed and can get infested with mites that can cause asthma symptoms in both people and pets.

_____ Wash dogs frequently.

_____ Consider removing carpeting or wood flooring if it has a strong animal urine odor.

Don't

_____ Lie on beds or sit on upholstered chairs belonging to people who may be allergic to your pet.

_____ Let your cat use the dirt crawl space off a basement as a litter box.

_____ Let your cat relieve itself on the "speedy-dry" powder (which is used on basement floors to absorb fuel-oil leaks).

► Pests

Do

_____ If there is a rank smell in a room

      _____ Put a box fan in a window on exhaust mode and close the other doors and windows in the room.

      _____ Cover all registers and grilles with foil and removable painters' tape while the fan is operating.

      _____ Cautiously sniff at electric outlets, light fixtures, and other openings in the ceiling or walls, even openings as small as a gap between a piece of wood trim and a wall.

      _____ If you find an opening that is particularly smelly, hire someone to open up that area of the wall or ceiling — either under containment or from the outside if possible — to find the pest nest. (Refer to Part I if mold rather than a pest nest is the culprit.)

      _____ Call a pest control operator (PCO) to help track down the location of and eradicate the pest infestation.

JEFF'S GEMS

When you set up negative pressure in a room by putting a box fan in a window on exhaust and closing all other doors and windows, air will flow from the wall and ceiling cavities into the room through construction gaps, electric outlets, light fixtures, and other openings. The strongest smell will emanate from those openings nearest the odor source — perhaps microbial growth in the HVAC system or mold growth or a pest infestation inside a wall or ceiling cavity. Refer to Part I, Dilemma 1F, "Heating and Cooling Systems," and Part I, Dilemma 2, "Confirmation and Remediation."

_____ If installing fiberglass insulation under an enclosed porch, cover the insulation with plywood.

    _____ Be sure there are no openings through which insects or rodents can enter. (Bees and mice like to nest in fiberglass.)

JEFF'S GEMS

Finger-sized tunnels in fiberglass insulation are often signs of rodent activity. If you look carefully around the tunnel, you can sometimes even see rodent droppings.

CONNIE'S COMMENTS

Yuck.

_____ Be alert for openings under porches, behind gutters, around soffits, at the bottom edge of siding, around bulkheads and entranceways, and in garages that can allow pests to enter.

_____ Using a mirror and a flashlight, check for openings at the bottom edge of siding, especially at stoops and additions.

_____ Use mortar to fill openings in masonry and wood, or expanding foam and 1/4-inch hardware cloth to fill openings in non-masonry walls.

_____ Make sure all gable and louver vents have intact screens.

_____ Have the wood structure in a new home treated with Timbor borate preservative to minimize mold growth and insect infestations (www.nisuscorp.com).

_____ Install a rain cap with an animal screen at the top of your chimney.

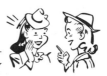

OTHER VOICES: A CASE STUDY

An old college friend of mine invited Connie and me over for dinner if I could solve an intermittent odor problem in his basement. He's a gourmet cook, so we accepted his offer with some excitement. At the top of the basement stairs I heard a periodic hissing noise and caught a whiff first of burned flesh and then of the sickening smell of a dead animal. His sons had just showered before we arrived, and water was dripping out of the water heater's vent pipe, hitting the hot draft-diverter below, and vaporizing in a puff of smoke, making that sound I'd heard from the top of the stairs. The water was forming from combustion gases, so that meant that either the vent pipe or the chimney was blocked.

My friend and I looked outside and couldn't see anything on top of the chimney that might be blocking the flue. We returned to the basement. I turned the water heater off and removed the vent pipe, which was heavier than I had anticipated. I took the pipe outside, held it in a vertical position and shook it into a bucket. Several charred bones fell out. I looked inside and could see a furry tail. I shook the pipe more vigorously and out fell a dead squirrel—cooked at the front half and rotting at the rear half.

The squirrel must have climbed down the chimney, crawled into the narrow heater vent pipe, and gotten stuck at the end of the pipe—a tragic death that could have been averted if my friend had had an animal screen at the top of the chimney.

Once the pipe was emptied of its odorous contents and reinstalled, the smell never returned. We got our free dinner, and thank God it was baked fish and not barbecued hamburger!

CONNIE'S COMMENTS

You should have seen Jeff's friend's face when the bones fell out of the vent pipe: He turned green. The whole situation was like a scene from the movie The Night of the Living Dead. *I'm surprised any of us could eat anything after that experience. And I have to say, I'll never look at a squirrel in quite the same way again.*

_____ Use metal rather than wooden bulkhead doors.

_____ Have an internal door inside the bulkhead.

_____ Set out sticky traps indoors near water and food sources to see if you have a cockroach infestation.

_____ To avoid attracting rodents, keep bird seed and dry pet food in sealed metal or plastic containers in your garage or basement.

_____ After a pest problem is eliminated, be sure the area of pest infestation is HEPA vacuumed (using a vacuum with high efficiency particulate arrestance filtration) and any urine-stained building materials disinfected and paint-sealed when dry.

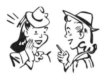 OTHER VOICES: A CASE STUDY

A couple noticed an intermittent, unpleasant odor in their family room, once a breezeway connecting the kitchen to the garage. When I went to the site, I didn't smell the odor, so I asked them to seal off the family room from the kitchen with plastic and run an exhaust fan in the window to reduce the air pressure in the room. The odor was then apparent, strongest at the floor opening around a pipe supplying hot water to a baseboard convector and smelling like rodent nesting.

There was a 3/4-inch hole under the siding at the outside corner of the garage, near the family room wall where I noted the odor. The back of the wall was in the garage, where the heat pipe for the family room was visible. I suggested to the owner that he make a hole in the drywall to look into that wall cavity. He was so anxious to solve the problem, however, that he grabbed a hammer and smashed through the drywall, right there and then. In the space he had opened up, we could see a trail of mouse droppings leading to the next wall bay. He smashed open that wall bay as well as the next wall bay.

The last wall bay he opened was full of foul-smelling sawdust, plant litter, and rodent droppings. The source of the smell was found at last!

_____ Keep grain and pet foods in tightly sealed containers to avoid flour moth infestations.

_____ Put wool clothing in sealed plastic boxes or bags to avoid wool moth infestations.

_____ If you smell a chemical odor in the basement or crawl space, find out if the building has ever been treated for termites.

     _____ If the answer is yes, find out if the chemical used was chlordane, a now-banned pesticide.

     _____ Confer with an IAQ professional about your options to control the chemical emissions.

Don't

_____ Have exposed fiberglass insulation under a porch or in a crawl space that is open to the exterior.

_____ Create nesting areas for rodents by keeping a lot of clutter on your garage floor.

_____ Have any garage wall or ceiling holes that open to cavities accessible to the habitable areas of your house.

_____ Spread pesticides on soil in a crawl space.

_____ Use excessive amounts of pesticides indoors, including bee and wasp sprays.

_____ Buy grain foods in a supermarket if you see a flour moth in them.

_____ Keep a wool rug that is infested with wool moths.

JEFF'S GEMS

Flour moths are about the same size as wool moths but are gray brown rather than gold colored. The moths metamorphose from white, worm-like larvae that eat grain. Sometimes you can see a flour moth fluttering around an open bin of grain in a supermarket. If a box of dry goods like rice, cereal, or even crackers is infested with wool-moth larvae, you may see white strings that look like spider webs in the box.

If you have a flour-moth infestation, you should throw away any opened dry goods. Remove all food from your shelves and thoroughly wash the shelves. The larvae can also hide behind paper labels and under jar caps, so your unopened dry goods as well as canned and jarred foods should be temporarily placed in a sealed storage bin. Check the bin and empty shelves every few days to see if any moths appear. If you find any, swat them. After the bin and shelves have been moth-free for at least two weeks, you can place your goods back on the shelves.

CONNIE'S COMMENTS

When Jeff and I were first married, we bought an oriental rug for our living room. It was a rich red color with gold threads, and we felt pretty lucky to have found it. About six months later, we discovered that the rug hadn't been such a great buy. The corner tucked under a chair, and thus not visible, was completely chewed up by moth larvae that were quivering all over the rug's surface. Talk about sickening!

For months after we got rid of that rug, we kept finding holes in wool sweaters, blankets, and scarves. I even found live moths nestled in fluffy wool balls stuck inside my carpet sweeper. We threw out a number of wool items we owned and encased the rest in plastic. That ended the moths' invasion, but it was a war from start to finish.

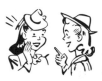

OTHER VOICES: A CASE STUDY

I've been finding shrew infestations in buildings more and more frequently in the last few years. Shrews are small, like mice, but eat meat like grubs and insects and supposedly have a pugnacious temperament. They defecate in a single location, and their fecal material piles up in a smelly cone or trail, which is particularly odoriferous in humid weather. The smell made by a few of these tiny creatures can drive people out of their homes, literally.

I was asked to look at one condo in a twelve-unit building that was a vacation home. The owner arrived for a two-week visit to find a smell in the

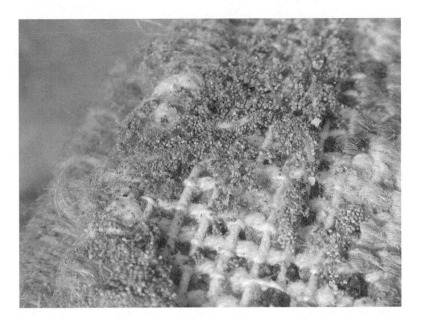

This is the back of our wool rug that was damaged by wool-moth larvae. You can see the backing with the missing fibers and the individual droppings from the creatures. Each dropping is about the size of a pinprick and has the color of the fiber that was consumed. *Jeffrey C. May*

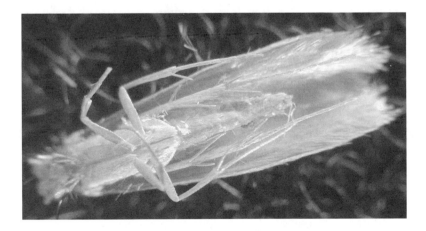

This straw-yellow wool moth was in our carpet. When I took the photo, the moth had been dead for a while, so its abdomen was shrunken. Like butterflies that emerge from cocoons, wool moths emerge from larvae. It is the larvae and not the adult moths that voraciously consume wool fibers. *Jeffrey C. May*

downstairs bedroom that was so strong he and his family couldn't use the room. In addition, the smell was traveling on air flows up into the unit above, where occupants were opening windows and spreading baking soda around to try to get rid of the odor. Eventually, through some sophisticated sleuthing that included setting up negative air pressure and collecting some of the fecal material to send to a lab for identification, I discovered that a shrew had moved into a wall cavity. I wasn't surprised to find a small hole at ground level at the exterior, right outside that corner of the smelly bedroom.

➤ For People with Allergies, Asthma, or Environmental Sensitivities

Do

_____ Send a vacuum-dust sample from a carpet to a lab to have the dust analyzed for dog, cat, roach, or dust mite allergens to which you may be sensitized.

_____ Replace any carpet formerly used by someone who owned a dog or cat if you or someone in your family is allergic to that animal.

      _____ Remember to replace carpeting on stairs and in hallways.

_____ If you or someone in your family is allergic to cats and you can't bring yourself to get rid of your pet cat, build an enclosure for the litter box that has a HEPA-filtered exhaust turned on by a motion detector.

_____ Ask your child's teacher not to have a pet in the classroom if your child is allergic to that animal.

_____ If you are chemically sensitive and have a pest problem, ask a pest control operator (PCO) to use borate pesticide.

_____ If paint fumes bother you, you can use a solution of Elmer's glue and water instead of paint to seal in irritating dust (approximately one to two parts water to one part glue).

Don't

_____ Use mothballs or pesticide sprays inside a building.

_____ Spread pesticides in the basement.

_____ Keep pet birds indoors. Their feathers are the source of all sorts of allergens.

_____ Allow dogs, cats, rabbits, hamsters, and other pets in bedrooms.

_____ Keep a fish tank in your bedroom. (Fish tank covers can acquire mite infestations.)

_____ Let people enter your house with pets if you are allergic to animal dander.

My Notes _____

_____

_____

_____

_____

_____

_____

_____

REMINDERS

1. *Be sure there are no openings on the outside of your home or in the garage that will allow pests to enter.*
2. *Don't buy grains in a supermarket in which you see a flour moth.*
3. *Keep wool items encased in plastic to help prevent wool moth infestations.*

WARNINGS

1. *Though it is rare, dogs and cats can have mites living in their fur. On the other hand, it is common for dog beds to be infested with mites.*
2. *Fish tank covers can acquire mite infestations, and allergens can become airborne when the cover is opened and closed. In addition, the frothing of the tank water can aerosolize bacterial and algal allergens.*
3. *Mothballs contain pesticide.*
4. *Exposed fiberglass insulation accessible from the exterior will become infested with mice, bees, or other pests.*

CONNIE'S COMMENTS

I'm not allergic to bees, but when I see one flying in my direction, I run away in terror. One summer several years ago, yellow jackets burrowed into a wall cavity next to our back-door entrance and built a nest. I stopped entering and exiting the house that way, because every time the door opened and closed, a few bees would zoom out of some hole and whiz around me in rage. We called a bee extermination company but had to wait a few days because they were booked. In the meantime, the yellow jackets found their way through wall cavities into our bedroom, where they buzzed up against the windows. Jeff didn't mind at all; he figured they wouldn't fly at night when he was asleep. He was probably right, but for me it was the last straw. I moved into the nearest Marriott and stayed there for three days until the exterminator removed the nest and rescued me.

RELEVANT RESOURCES

Laboratories That Sell Test Kits and Analyze Dust Samples from Carpets and Other Surfaces

Aerotech Labs, Phoenix, AZ (800-651-4802, www.aerotechpk.com).

DACI Laboratory, Johns Hopkins University Asthma and Allergy Center, Baltimore, MD (800-344-3224, www.hopkinsmedicine.org/allergy/daci/index.html).

Northeast Laboratory, Winslow, ME (800-244-8378, www.nelabservices.com).

Products

Boracare and Timbor: These products minimize mold and insect infestations for people who are chemically sensitive. If in doubt, use Timbor. In most states, these products must be applied by professionals. The Nisus Corporation in Rockford, TN (800-264-0870, http://nisuscorp.com) manufactures these products.

Cockroach, dust mite, and pet allergen test kits: DACI Laboratory, Johns Hopkins

University Asthma and Allergy Center, Baltimore, MD (800-344-3224, www.hopkinsmedicine.org/allergy/daci/index.html).

Pet allergen test kit: Aerotech Labs, Phoenix, AZ (800-651-4802, www.aerotechpk .com).

A Publication

Integrated Pest Management (IPM) in Schools, Environmental Protection Agency (www.epa/gov/pesticides/ipm/).

F. RENOVATION AND CONSTRUCTION

_____ There are irritating paint fumes and construction dust in an area undergoing renovation.

_____ There's a funny smell in my house.

In what room or rooms? _____

What's the smell like? _____

_____ I'm worried there may be asbestos in some of the construction materials

    _____ In insulation wrap around old heat pipes or ducts.

    _____ In old resilient tile flooring in a basement.

    _____ Somewhere else _____

_____ I'm worried there may be lead paint in my house.

_____ I have other concerns. _____

_____

_____

_____

➤ Renovation

Do

_____ To prevent the spread of vapors and particulates, isolate work areas by setting up containment.

    _____ Close and cover with plastic any doorways leading to other spaces.

    _____ Use tacky mats (www.pro-tect.com) at containment exits to prevent dust spreading into habitable areas on workers' shoes.

    _____ Use an exhaust fan to create negative air pressure.

JEFF'S GEMS

To set up containment, you need to isolate the work area from the rest of the house. Doors and other openings leading from the work area to the rest of the house should be closed and sealed by covering them with plastic. A fan should be used on exhaust to blow air out of the work area and thus reduce the air pressure. Air then flows through gaps and cracks into the work area from adjacent habitable spaces, rather than vice versa.

_____ Keep the air conditioning or heat off whenever possible, to prevent contamination of the air duct system.

_____ Install supplementary filter materials over air supplies and returns whether or not the heating or cooling system will be operated.

_____ Filters in the HVAC (heating, ventilation, and air conditioning) system may have to be changed more frequently.

_____ Use only new drop cloths, because old ones may contain lead paint dust or allergens from previous jobs.

_____ Remove personal possessions from the work area or seal them in plastic.

_____ After the renovation project is complete, HEPA vacuum (using a vacuum with high efficiency particulate arrestance filtration) all surfaces and then damp-wipe solid surfaces.

Don't

_____ Allow dusty work such as sanding drywall, sawing wood, or sweeping floors to take place when a hot-air or air conditioning system is operating and the ducts are unprotected by filter material.

_____ Apply creosote-containing preservatives to interior or basement wood.

► Construction Materials

Do

_____ Determine if a vinyl product such as a window shade or insect screen is emitting (off-gassing) an annoying chemical odor by removing the item from the room to see if the odor goes away.

_____ Replace off-gassing vinyl insect screens with aluminum insect screens.

_____ Replace any ceiling tiles that have a strong smell.

    _____ Cover furniture and carpets to protect them from ceiling-tile dust, which can contain fiberglass or rodent droppings.

_____ Turn off all the lights, then turn them on one by one to see if any is the source of a dead-fish odor.

_____ If you think walls or ceiling may be emitting an odor

    _____ Air out the room.

    _____ Try the paper-towel test to find the source of an odor. (See Part I, Dilemma 1H, "Hotels and Automobiles.")

    _____ If it appears as though the paint is the source of the odor, contact the paint manufacturer and have a representative visit.

    _____ Wash the offending surface with a cleaner suited for the purpose (preferably unfragranced).

    _____ It those steps don't help, buy an alcohol-based, shellac primer/sealer paint like BIN, available in many paint, building supply, and hardware stores; paint the surface and repeat the paper-towel test.

    _____ If all else fails, you can replace the drywall or have Dennyfoil (a paper-aluminum foil laminate) and then new drywall installed over the old wall or ceiling.

_____ If you think that hardwood floors are emitting an odor

    _____ Try the paper-towel test to find the source of an odor. (See Part I, Dilemma 1H, "Hotels and Automobiles.")

    _____ Wash the floor with a suitable cleaner (unfragranced if possible).

    _____ Cover the floor with aluminum foil or Dennyfoil to minimize off-gassing and see if the odor stops bothering you.

    _____ Consider refinishing the floor.

➤ Asbestos

Do

_____ Have older (pre-1980) tiles, particularly if they are 9 inches by 9 inches, checked for asbestos.

_____ Hire a qualified professional to test insulation for asbestos.

_____ Hire a professional remediator to remove asbestos-containing materials under containment.

      _____ Research state and federal regulations regarding asbestos remediation.

Don't

_____ Disturb material you think may contain asbestos.

_____ Remediate asbestos unless you are trained to do so and allowed to do so by law.

OTHER VOICES: A CASE STUDY

A family was considering buying a house with asbestos-cement shingles on the roof. Concerned that asbestos might be present in the soil outside the house, they sent samples of the soil and debris from the gutter to a lab for analysis. The content of asbestos varied between 10% and 25% in all the samples. The family purchased the property and then hired a company to remediate, including removing the asbestos-containing roof tiles. This work had to be done under containment, so the house was tented under plastic. Unfortunately, the remediators left the house windows open during the remediation work, and asbestos contaminated the entire interior of the house, resulting in a remediation cost well in excess of the original estimate.

► Lead Paint

Do

_____ Ask people to take their shoes off at your door if you think the soil outside your house may contain lead paint dust.

_____ To test for lead

      _____ Purchase a lead test, available at many hardware and building supply stores.

_____ Or send a sample of the material you think contains lead to a lab.

_____ Or have a qualified professional test paint inside your home for lead.

_____ Send a sample of soil from the ground around your foundation to a lab for lead testing.

_____ Hire a professional to encapsulate or remove lead paint under containment.

_____ Research state and federal regulations regarding lead abatement.

Don't

_____ Use drop cloths indoors if they may have been used (indoors or outdoors) when lead paint was scraped or sanded.

_____ Sand lead paint.

_____ Remove lead paint unless you are trained to do so and allowed to do so by law.

_____ Let your children play in the dirt close to the foundation outside your house if you think it may contain lead paint chips or dust.

OTHER VOICES: A CASE STUDY

A young couple owned a condo in a hundred-year-old Victorian single family home that had been divided into two units. When they had their first child they found that the condo was too small, so they decided to put it on the market and look for a bigger home. They did some redecorating because they wanted to get the best price they could for their condo. They were in the process of sanding the woodwork to prepare it for painting when they received an excellent offer. As part of the pre-purchase inspection the prospective buyer had lead testing done in the unit. High levels of lead were found in all the rooms, including in the baby's crib and on the baby's toys. The paint that the young couple had sanded contained lead, and the dust was all over their home. Needless to say, they were ordered to immediately evacuate the premises.

➤ For People with Allergies, Asthma, or Environmental Sensitivities

Do

_____ Confer with an IAQ professional if you can't figure out the source of a smell or why you sneeze, cough, or have watery eyes in a particular room.

_____ Ask renovators to use your HEPA vacuum (a machine with high efficiency particulate arrestance filtration) and new drop cloths.

_____ If sensitized to paint off-gassing, test any paint you plan to use on a piece of wood outdoors and see if the paint film, once dry, is a problem for you. (See Part II, Dilemma 3B, "Other Rooms and Their Contents.")

_____ If you are sensitive to solvents, test a floor finish first on a piece of wood outdoors to see if the finish, once dry, is a problem for you.

_____ Highly sensitized individuals may have to relocate temporarily while renovation work is ongoing.

_____ If you are traveling and are sensitive to dust and paint solvent, ask if renovation or remodeling work is going on in a hotel before you book a room there.

_____ Eliminate the cedar in a cedar closet or cover the walls with Dennyfoil and drywall.

Don't

_____ Use paint with added mildewcide indoors.

_____ Use fragrant, exotic wood such as Brazilian cherry for floors if you are chemically sensitive.

My Notes _____

_____
_____
_____
_____
_____
_____
_____
_____

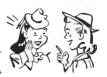

OTHER VOICES: Q & A

Q: We built a new house. I'm very sensitive to odors, so we took great care in selecting products and decided not to have any wall-to-wall carpeting. The first floor is tiled, and yet I still can't stay in the house for any length of time without feeling disoriented and experiencing brain fog. My husband and daughter don't seem to have any problems in the house. What could have gone wrong?

A: It's not surprising that you are the only one in your family who is symptomatic in the home, as it's often the case that only one person in a group is sensitized to the environment.

You may have made all the right choices for building materials, but occasionally there are problems with individual batches of construction products. We've seen paints that produced sulfur-like odors, joint compound that produced a chemical odor (possibly from added fungicide), vinyl window frames that smelled like mold, exotic wood flooring that off-gassed a cedar-like odor, ceiling tiles that smelled like vomit, and light fixtures that smelled like dead fish. Carefully and methodically try to locate the source of the odor by cautiously sniffing every surface. Don't be embarrassed to crawl around and look foolish. Be as thorough as you can; you never know where the source may be located.

If you are still stymied, ask an IAQ professional to investigate.

REMINDERS

1. *A space undergoing renovation should be isolated from other areas of the building.*
2. *Abatement of lead paint and asbestos-containing materials must be done by trained professionals who set up containment and follow applicable state and federal regulations.*

WARNINGS

1. *Bacteria that contaminate some ceiling tiles produce butyric acid — a chemical that smells like vomit. Such tiles should be replaced.*
2. *The nylon electrical insulator in the Edison base of some light fixtures smells like dead fish when heated.*
3. *Mildewcides and fungicides in paint can be irritating to those who are sensitized.*

RELEVANT RESOURCES

Laboratories That Sell Test Kits and Analyze Dust Samples

Aerotech Labs, Phoenix, AZ (800-651-4802, www.aerotechpk.com).
DACI Laboratory, Johns Hopkins University Asthma and Allergy Center, Baltimore, MD (800-344-3224, www.hopkinsmedicine.org/allergy/daci/index.html).
Envirologix in Portland, ME (866-408-4597, http://envirologix.com) also sells test kits for mycotoxins.
Northeast Laboratory, Winslow, ME (800-244-8378, www.nelabservices.com).

Products

Dennyfoil: A paper–aluminum foil laminate that can be used to temporarily cover surfaces. Denny Wholesale (561-750-3705, www.dennywholesale.com).
Lead test: Available in many hardware and building supply stores.
Pro-Tect, a self-adhering, clear plastic: Pro-Tect Associates, Inc. (800-545-0826, www.pro-tect.com).

Publications

The Healthy House, John Bower. Bloomington, IN: Healthy House Institute, 2001.
IAQ Guidelines for Occupied Buildings under Construction. Chantilly, VA: Sheet Metal and Air Conditioning Contractors' National Association, Inc., 1995.

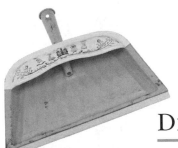

DILEMMA 4

Everyday Cleaning

_____ The vacuum cleaner has an unpleasant smell when it's being used.

_____ The broom closet has a rotten odor.

_____ Surfaces smell bad after they've been cleaned.

_____ Scented cleaning products are used that I find irritating.

_____ I have other concerns. _____

_____

_____

_____

_____

JEFF'S GEMS

Cleaning and maintenance practices should reduce potential sources of indoor air quality problems. Unfortunately the opposite is sometimes the case. A sponge or mop contaminated with bacterial growth can make surfaces or a broom closet smell rotten. Fragranced cleaning products can be irritating to those who are sensitized. (Fragrances cover up smells and should not be necessary if surfaces are cleaned properly and kept clean.) Vacuum cleaners without HEPA (high efficiency particulate arrestance) filters can spew out allergens in their exhaust, and dust heated in a vacuum motor can create annoying burned odors.

Do

_____ Replace sponges and mop heads regularly.

_____ Run a sponge that smells rotten through your dishwasher along with the dirty dishes.

_____ With a solution of one tablespoon of ammonia or one teaspoon of baking soda in a cup of water, clean a surface that has acquired a rotten smell from being wiped with a dirty sponge. (First test a spot to be sure that the solution will not damage the finish.)

_____ Consider using rags instead of a sponge; wash the rags frequently.

_____ Always check the instructions and labels on cleaning products (even if organic).

    _____ Avoid mixing chemicals that may interact adversely.

    _____ Never mix or use bleach- and ammonia-containing products together.

    _____ If possible, store bleach and ammonia in separate, child-safe cabinets.

_____ Open a window for fresh air when using a strong-smelling cleaner in a small room.

_____ To minimize chemical aerosols, use wipes containing cleaning solution rather than spray cleaners.

_____ Use a HEPA-filtered vacuum or a central vacuum system, but only if it vents to the exterior.

    _____ Change the filters according to the manufacturer's directions.

CONNIE'S COMMENTS

Vacuum cleaners with HEPA filters are expensive but worth the cost. We bought our first one years ago when our son, who has asthma and dust allergies, was a little boy. He used to cough and sneeze whenever we vacuumed (the apple doesn't fall far from the tree), but that stopped when we started using a HEPA vacuum. The first one we bought was a commercial unit and felt as if it weighed a hundred pounds, so it was difficult to lug around. Newer canister models are much lighter and easier to use.

_____ Have rugs and wall-to-wall carpets professionally cleaned.

_____ Use steam vapor to reduce allergens and kill insect pests in cushioned furniture and carpeting. (See Part I, Dilemma 1A, "My Basement.")

_____ Follow the manufacturer's directions carefully for safe use.

_____ Spot-check some of the material first to make sure the steam does not cause any damage.

_____ To treat a rug with steam vapor, suspend or hang the rug away from a wall or any varnished surface, including wood floors.

_____ Where appropriate for the fabric, dry-clean clothing to kill mites and destroy mite allergens.

Don't

_____ Use products that contain ammonia and products that contain bleach at the same time.

_____ Use a steam-vapor machine to clean area rugs that lie on finished hardwood floors.

_____ Depend on an air purifier to clean the air if the sources of contaminants and irritants have not been removed.

_____ Regularly use an air purifier that produces ozone (an irritating gas) if occupants are present.

➤ For People with Allergies, Asthma, or Environmental Sensitivities

Do

_____ Air out dry-cleaned clothing before hanging the items in a closet or putting them away in a bureau drawer.

_____ In a building with operable windows, HEPA vacuum carpets more frequently than usual during the pollen season.

_____ Make sure anyone you hire to clean your home uses your HEPA-filtered or central vacuum system and unfragranced cleaning products.

_____ If you have dust allergies, wear a NIOSH (National Institute of Occupational Safety and Health) N95 mask while vacuuming.

Don't

_____ Let anyone clean your house with any other vacuum other than your HEPA vacuum.

_____ Let anyone use a non-HEPA-filtered shop vacuum for cleaning in your home, even during renovation.

My Notes _____

_____

_____

_____

_____

OTHER VOICES: Q & A

Q: I moved into an apartment where the previous tenant had two cats. I'm allergic to cats, so I had the carpets cleaned. I still sneeze whenever I come home from work. I purchased a portable air purifier, hoping that this would clean the air. It actually made it worse. Now I'm sneezing more and sometimes my eyes water. What can I do, other than move?

A: Some air purifiers are designed to kick up dust with the exhaust air flow so that, in theory, the dust can then be removed by the purifier's filter. Unfortunately more dust is usually disturbed and aerosolized than removed, which is probably why you are feeling worse when the air purifier is operating. I suspect that the carpet is the source of most of the allergen. Try raising the machine up off the floor to see if this makes a difference.

You don't describe how you had the carpet cleaned. Typical steam cleaning may not eliminate enough allergens. Treatment with steam vapor can denature (destroy) allergens without introducing chemicals or excessive moisture into the carpet, but always check first with the carpet manufacturer about using steam vapor, because the high temperature may damage the carpet fibers. If you continue to suffer symptoms, the carpet may have to be removed. For the moment, however, you can cover the carpet with Pro-tect, an adhesive film, and then, if you like, cover the Pro-tect with some area rugs.

If you have hot-water heat with baseboard convectors, these should also be HEPA vacuumed and the fin tubing cleaned with steam vapor, because these surfaces may be coated with dust containing cat allergen.

If all these steps don't help, you may have to live in another apartment.

REMINDERS

1. *Avoid using heavily scented cleaning products.*
2. *Use cleaning wipes instead of spray cleaners.*

WARNINGS

1. *When bleach and ammonia are mixed together, the toxic gas chloramine is formed.*
2. *Ozone gas is an irritant.*
3. *Even so-called "organic" cleaning agents are chemicals and can cause irritation.*

RELEVANT RESOURCES

Institutes that Train Cleaning Professionals

Restoration Industry Association (RIA), Columbia, MD (800-272-7012, www.ascr.org).

Institute of Inspection, Cleaning and Restoration Certification (IICRC), Vancouver, WA (800-835-4624, www.certifiedcleaners.org).

Restoration Consultants, Sacramento, CA (888-617-3266, www.restcon.com).

Products

Carpet covering (self-adhering clear plastic): Pro-tect Associates, Inc., Northfield, IL (800-545-0826, www.pro-tect.com).

HEPA vacuum cleaner: Available in many home supply stores as well as online. (See www.miele.com.)

NIOSH N95 mask: Available in most hardware and building supply stores. Brands include 3M #8210 and Gerson #1710.

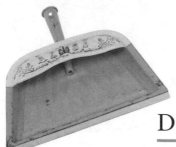

DILEMMA 5

Testing

———— I want to have a space tested for contaminants.
———— I have a testing report I don't understand.
———— A testing report says that the building's air is clean, and yet I'm still experiencing symptoms.
———— I have other concerns. ————————————————
————————————————————————————————
————————————————————————————————

JEFF'S GEMS

A few tests building occupants can use are available in hardware and building supply stores or can be purchased directly from testing laboratories. Most tests for VOC (volatile organic compound) contaminants, however, are done only by IAQ professionals.

Do

———— Find out what IAQ tests you can do yourself.

———— For carbon monoxide: Buy a digital readout, plug-in carbon monoxide detector, available in many hardware and building supply stores.

———— For formaldehyde: Get a passive formaldehyde test kit from a testing lab.

_____ For radon: Buy a passive radon test kit from a building supply or hardware store.

_____ Confer with an IAQ professional and/or an appropriately trained or experienced environmental physician on the meaning and implications of a test result or an IAQ testing report.

Don't

_____ Use any chemicals, solvents, pesticides, cleaners, paints, nail polish or remover, or spray fragrances before or during a test for VOCs.

➤ For People with Allergies, Asthma, or Environmental Sensitivities

Do

_____ If you are still having health problems indoors after the building has been tested for VOCs and the results are negative, ask that the area be retested during a time when you generally experience symptoms.

JEFF'S GEMS

Concentrations of chemicals that affect a chemically sensitive person are usually below the limit of detection of most testing methods. If you are chemically sensitive and are having symptoms, it doesn't matter that test results for VOCs are reassuring. Your body is the best indicator of the presence of potentially irritating chemicals.

My Notes _____

_____

_____

_____

_____

_____

_____

REMINDER

Confer with an IAQ professional if you do not understand the results of an IAQ test report.

WARNING

Based on the results of an IAQ test you did yourself, don't make drastic decisions such as evacuating a house. Have an IAQ professional test again for verification. The only exception is a carbon monoxide detector that warns of dangerously elevated levels of this lethal gas. In this case, you should leave the house immediately.

RELEVANT RESOURCES

Laboratories That Sell Test Kits

Aerotech Labs, Phoenix, AZ (800-651-4802, www.aerotechpk.com).

DACI Laboratory, Johns Hopkins University Asthma and Allergy Center, Baltimore, MD (800-344-3224, www.hopkinsmedicine.org/allergy/daci/index.html).

Envirologix, Portland, ME (866-408-4597, http://envirologix.com) also sells test kits for pesticide residues and mycotoxins.

Northeast Laboratory, Winslow, ME (800-244-8378, www.nelabservices.com).

Organizations

American Conference of Governmental Industrial Hygienists, Cincinnati, OH (513-742-2020, www.acgih.org).

American Industrial Hygiene Association, Fairfax, VA (743-849-8888, www.aiha.org).

Products

Carbon monoxide monitor: NSI 3000 low-level CO monitor from National Comfort Institute, Sheffield Lake, OH (800-633-7058, www .nationalcomfortinstitute.com).

Formaldehyde test kit: SKC Inc., Eighty Four, PA (800-752-8472, www.skcinc.com).

Ozone gas passive indicator: Ozone Watch, IAQ Air (877-715-4247, www.iqair .com).

Radon Test: Alpha-Trak, National Safety Products, Inc. (877-412-3600, http:// testproducts.com). Also available in many building supply and hardware stores.

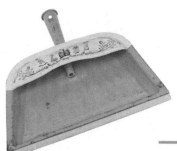

Conclusion

CONNIE'S FINAL COMMENTS

I must admit, sometimes my eyes glaze over when Jeff goes on and on about mold spores and dust mite fecal pellets and pet dander and excessive relative humidity . . . and . . . and . . . But in our own home, we practice what he preaches.

Jeff has a lot of allergies: to mold, pollen, and dogs — not to mention all the food allergies he faces. And our two children have asthma. After our son suffered a life-threatening asthma attack and was hospitalized for a week, we tried changing the conditions in our home to better control his symptoms. Jeff took dust samples of our bedding and carpeting, and sampled the air coming from some of our heat registers. He found evidence of dust mites and mold. We put allergen-control encasings on all our mattresses and pillows. We got rid of a rug and our feather quilt. We had the heating system cleaned. (We eventually moved into a house with radiator heat.) All these steps helped. Both our children still experienced symptoms, but they didn't seem to experience them as often or with such severity — at least at home. And Jeff felt better, too.

So it's no surprise that helping people take charge of conditions in their environment so they can improve or guard their health became one of the biggest commitments of Jeff's life. We hope this book has helped you. If it has, please encourage other people to use it in the same way: as a practical guide and a record of progress made improving the quality of air in a home. And let us know how things are going. We are genuinely interested, we promise.

Additional Resources

Inclusion in the list that follows or in the resource lists at the end of certain sections of the book does not constitute an endorsement by the authors or the publisher. The list is intended to help readers gather information and make up their own minds as to which organizations, labs, products, and publications may help them deal with their indoor environmental questions and concerns.

ORGANIZATIONS

American Academy of Allergy, Asthma and Immunology, Milwaukee, WI (414-272-6071, www.aaaai.org).

American Academy of Environmental Medicine, Wichita, KS (316-684-5500, www.aaem.com).

American Academy of Pediatrics, Elk Grove Village, IL (847-434-4000, www.aap.org).

American Board of Medical Specialties, Evanston, IL (847-491-9091), www.abms.org).

American Indoor Air Quality Association, Rockville, MD (301-231-8388, www.iaqa.org).

American Lung Association, New York, NY (800-586-4872, www.lungusa.org).

American Public Health Association, Washington, DC (202-777-APHA, www.apha.org).

Asthma and Allergy Foundation of America, Washington, DC (202-466-7642, www.aafa.org).

Center for Health, Environment, and Justice, Falls Church, VA (703-237-2249, www.chej.org).

Centers for Disease Control and Prevention, National Center for Environmental Health, Atlanta, GA (800-311-3435, www.cdc.gov/).

Children's Environmental Health Network, Washington, DC, and Berkeley, CA (202-543-4033 and 510-526-0081, www.cehn.org).

Connecticut Foundation for Environmentally Safe Schools (www.pollutionfreeschools.org, information@pollutionfreeschools.org).

Healthy Kids: The Key to Basics, Newton, MA (617-965-9637, www.healthy-kids.info/aboutus.lasso).

Healthy Schools Network, Inc., Albany, NY (518-462-0632, 212-482-0204, www.healthyschools.org).

Indoor Air Quality Information Clearing House (800-438-4318). The EPA's indoor air quality information hotline.

National Center for Healthy Housing, Columbia, MD (410-992-0712, www.centerforhealthyhousing.org).

National Institute of Occupational Safety and Health, Atlanta, GA (404-639-3534, 800-311-3435, www.cdc.gov/niosh/homepage.html).

New York City Department of Health and Mental Hygiene (http://home2.nyc.gov/html/doh/html/home/home.shtml).

Occupational Safety and Health Administration, U.S. Department of Labor, Washington, DC (866-4-USA-DOL, www.osha.gov).

U.S. Environmental Protection Agency (EPA), National Center for Environmental Publications, Cincinnati, OH (800-490-9198, www.epa.gov/iaq).

PUBLICATIONS

An Introduction to Indoor Air Quality, Environmental Protection Agency (www.epa.gov/iaq/ia-intro.html).

Causes of Indoor Air Quality Problems in Schools, Charlene W. Bayer, Sidney A. Crow, and John Fischer. The Energy Division, Oak Ridge National Laboratory for the U.S. Department of Energy, January 1999.

Casualties of Progress: Personal Histories from the Chemically Sensitive, Alison Johnson, ed. Brunswick, ME: MCS Information Exchange, 2000.

"Damp Indoor Spaces and Health," Committee on Damp Indoor Spaces and Health, Institute of Medicine, National Academy of Sciences, 2004 (www.iom.edu/CMS/3793/4703/20223.aspx).

"Fungi and Indoor Air Quality," Sandra V. McNeel, DVM, and Richard A. Kreustzer, MD. *Health and Environmental Digest* 10, no. 2 (May/June 1996): 9-12.

Green Guide for Health Care, convened by the Center for Maximum Potential Building Systems, sponsored by Hospitals for a Healthy Environment (H2E) and the New York State Energy Research and Development Authority (NYSERDA). Funding provided by the Merck Family Fund (www.gghc.org).

"Guidance for Clinicians on the Recognition and Management of Health Effects Related to Mold Exposure and Moisture Indoors," Eileen Storey et al. Farmington, CT: University of Connecticut Health Center, 2004 (www.oehc.edu/clinser/MOLD%20Guide.pdf).

Guidelines for Environmental Infection Control in Health-Care Facilities, Lynne Sehulster and Raymond Y.W. Chinn, Center for Disease Control and Prevention (www.cdc.gov/mmwr/preview/mmwrhtml/rr5210a1.htm).

Handbook of Pediatric Environmental Health, Ruth Ann Etzel and Sophie J. Balk, eds. Elk Grove, IL: American Academy of Pediatrics, 1999.

How to Operate Your Home, Tom Feiza, "Mr. Fix-It," Inc. New Berlin, WI: Mr. Fix-It Press, 2006. (262-786-7878, www.howtooperateyourhome.com). Every homeowner should have this book.

Indoor Air Quality and HVAC Systems, David W. Bearg. Boca Raton, FL: Lewis Publishers, 1993.

"Indoor Air Quality Tools for Schools," the EPA's action kit, which offers parents and educators a practical plan for solving IAQ problems in school buildings. Available through the Indoor Air Quality Clearing House (800-438-4318; www.epa.gov/iaq).

Mold Remediation in Schools and Commercial Buildings, #402-K-01-001, Environmental Protection Agency, March 2001 (www.epa.gov/mold/mold _ remediation.html).

The Mold Survival Guide: For Your Home and for Your Health, Jeffrey C. May and Connie L. May. Baltimore, MD: Johns Hopkins University Press, 2004.

"Molds, Toxic Molds, and Indoor Air Quality," Pamela J. Davis, *CRB Note* 8, no. 1 (March 2001) (www.library.ca.gov/crb/01/notes/v8n1.pdf).

My House Is Killing Me! The Home Guide for Families with Allergies and Asthma, Jeffrey C. May, Baltimore, MD: Johns Hopkins University Press, 2001.

My Office Is Killing Me! The Sick Building Survival Guide, Jeffrey C. May. Baltimore, MD: Johns Hopkins University Press, 2006.

"Policy Statement Toxic Effects of Indoor Molds," American Academy of Pediatrics, 101, no. 4 (April 1998): 712-714 (www.aehf.com/articles/APMmold.htm).

A SERVICE

May Indoor Air Investigations LLC in Tyngsboro, MA, investigates mold, moisture, odor, and indoor air quality problems throughout the country (978-649-1055, www.mayindoorair.com).

Index

84, 93–98; for ozone, 175; for pet allergens, 158–59; for radon, 135, 173; resources for, 174–75; for volatile organic compounds, 172, 173. *See also* carbon monoxide detectors; gas detectors; radon
Therma-Stor Santa Fe, 18–19, 24
toilets, 114, 115. *See also* bathrooms

ultrasonic tank-testing, 143
urea-formaldehyde glue, 124, 125

vacuum cleaners, 104, 167. *See also* HEPA vacuum
vapor barriers, 15–16
ventilation: of attics, 34–36, 41; of bathrooms, 115; of crawl spaces, 14; of dryers, 56, 117, 138; of heating equipment, 138–39
vinyl products, 42, 43, 117, 160–61
volatile organic compounds (VOCs), 125, 172, 173

walls, mold on, 52–53
washing machines. *See* laundry areas
water heaters, 77, 78
water stains, 60
Wizard Stick, to track air flows, 130, 135
wood stoves, 128, 129, 130–31
wood surfaces, 101
wool moths, 154, 155

About the Authors

Jeffrey C. May has put his nose and air-sampling instruments into thousands of homes, schools, and offices. And with his microscope he has looked at over 25,000 air and dust samples to hunt for mold spores, dust mite droppings, pollen, bacteria, yeast, and animal dander. He suffered through three years of graduate school in organic chemistry at Harvard, for which he received a master's degree. He is the author of *My House Is Killing Me! The Home Guide for Families with Allergies and Asthma* and *My Office Is Killing Me! The Sick Building Survival Guide,* as well as co-author of *The Mold Survival Guide: For Your Home and for Your Health.* Principal scientist of May Indoor Air Investigations LLC in Tyngsboro, Massachusetts, Jeff lectures on indoor air quality and investigates building problems all over the country.

Connie L. May spent twenty-eight exhausting years as a high school English teacher, admissions officer, and college counselor before joining May Indoor Air Investigations LLC and becoming co-author of *The Mold Survival Guide: For Your Home and for Your Health.* She is also co-author of a textbook series on expository and creative writing and author of two (as yet) unpublished novels that have nothing to do with mold or indoor air quality.